THIRTY DAYS
TO BETTER
NUTRITION

VIRGINIA ARONSON, R.D., M.S.

Department of Nutrition
Harvard University
School of Public Health
Boston, Massachusetts

Foreword by
Fredrick J. Stare, M.D.,
Professor Emeritus,
Harvard's Department of Nutrition

Illustrated by David Bastille

DOUBLEDAY & COMPANY, INC.
GARDEN CITY, NEW YORK
1984

To my father who is moderate
in all things.

First Published in 1983 by John Wright · PSG Inc.,
545 Great Road, Littleton, Massachusetts 01460, U.S.A.
John Wright & Sons Ltd., 823–825 Bath Road,
Bristol BS4 5NU, England

Library of Congress Cataloging in Publication Data
Aronson, Virginia.
Thirty days to better nutrition.
Originally published as: A practical guide to
optimal nutrition. Boston: J. Wright-PSG, 1983.
Bibliography: p.
1. Nutrition. I. Title.
QP141.A694   1984   613.2   84-10264
ISBN 0-385-19418-8

Foreword

by Fredrick J. Stare, M.D., founder and former chairman,
Harvard's Department of Nutrition (currently Professor Emeritus), Boston, Massachusetts

Today's health-conscious public is constantly clamoring for new dieting ideas and answers to everyday nutrition concerns: how to lose weight—and keep it off—without the pain of physical and emotional deprivation, tips on dining out without diet destruction, incorporating exercise into a busy lifestyle, eating for the sportsman and woman, facts on food additives, vitamins and nutrition supplements, "health foods" and "junk foods," sugar, salt, cholesterol, alcohol, vegetarianism—the list goes on and on.

Confused by the mixed messages of media hype, the lures of food supplement salespersons, and the scare tactics of food activists and extremists, the typical American consumer needs professional guidance in order to be able to confidently enjoy the well-balanced diet which is so readily available.

As a physician, professor and founder of Harvard's Department of Nutrition, I have spent the last few decades both trying to educate the nutritionally naive public by providing basic dietary guidance, and attempting to combat the ever-increasing factions of pseudonutritionists and fad diet gurus. I find my task to be increasingly difficult, as scientists steadily reveal greater insight into the intricacies of nutrition, while the medically unprofessional and nutritionally negligent elements of our society continue to take advantage of public hopes, fears and gullibility by distorting the evidence to meet their own, often selfish needs. Thus, despite the current existence of the most safe, affordable, delicious and nutritious food supply ever available to any society, many Americans are convinced that they must be undernourished, so they waste billions of dollars each year in misguided quests for optimal nutrition. Health food stores have mushroomed into a booming industry, the mega-sales of nutritional supplements continue to expand, the so-called "natural" market includes everything from beer and chips to cosmetics, and a new celebrity diet/exercise book hits the top of the best sellers charts nearly every month. Obviously, the path ahead for concerned nutrition educators is a long and difficult one, littered with public confusion, media exaggeration, and pseudonutritional misdirection.

It is always a pleasant surprise for me to come across a source of sensible nutrition information: An occasional well-researched television special, a radio talk show featuring a reliable professional, or a scientifically valid magazine piece by a responsible journalist can really serve to brighten my outlook on the future of nutrition education. Perhaps even more encouraging—and certainly more rare—is the discovery of a well-researched, well-written, comprehensible nutrition book by a reliable, responsible professional. This book is one of these inspiring, infrequent finds.

Thirty Days to Better Nutrition provides readers with up-to-date nutrition facts in an easy-to-read and palatable format. It is a thirty-day program designed so that even nutritional neophytes can learn to incorporate important dietary concepts into their own individual lifestyles. *Thirty Days to Better Nutrition* also provides nutrition educators—dietitians, nutritionists, doctors, nurses, and other health professionals—with a source of basic nutrition information from which to derive their own lesson plans, a book they can recommend to students, patients, and clients.

Thirty Days to Better Nutrition was written by one of the best and hardest-working research assistants I have ever had, and I feel privileged to write this Foreword to heartily recommend the book to all. It is currently on the Recommended Reading List that I and one or more of my associates have provided to the public for many years, and which is updated two or three times a year. It should be on your own reading list, and in your library as well.

Fredrick J. Stare, M.D.
August, 1984

Contents

Introduction

The New York *Times* best sellers list consistently includes at least one title on nutrition or diet. Bookstore shelves are overflowing with a variety of paperbacks on eating and health. Newspapers and magazines constantly offer articles on food and fitness. Unfortunately, much of the nutrition information presented to the public—in books, newspapers, magazines, and on radio and television—is misleading.

So what can the uninformed consumer do? How can the public differentiate between scientific fact and nutrition nonsense?

The only answer for the confused layperson is to obtain some usable nutrition know-how from knowledgeable, well-trained professionals. *Thirty Days to Better Nutrition* can provide the nutritionally naïve reader with the basics of nutrition, the newest facts on diet and health, and tips for improving nutritional status. And *Thirty Days to Better Nutrition* presents this information in an easy-to-read and practical manner, enabling readers to incorporate this new information into their individual lifestyles.

After conducting a number of weight control clinics, counseling hundreds of nutrition clients, and presenting nutrition workshops to a variety of audiences, I became convinced that a book like *Thirty Days to Better Nutrition* was desperately needed and consciously desired by the American public. So many of my clients and such a large majority of my audiences asked me to recommend a comprehensible and usable nutrition text that I finally realized in despair that someone had to write such a book...and soon. My path was laid out before me!

Thirty Days to Better Nutrition has been written so that readers can gradually incorporate important nutrition concepts into their individual living patterns. The basics of balanced diet, weight control, and healthful eating will gradually become part of each reader's individual lifestyle, as he or she reads and participates in a different chapter each day. After all, eating is one of life's greatest pleasures, and a daily necessity. Why not eat right and enjoy it, so that both diet and overall health can be optimized?

Thirty Days to Better Nutrition can also be utilized in the classroom setting, as it is organized in such a way that class lesson plans can easily be composed around the daily nutrition information. Nursing, medical, and dental students, nutrition nonprofessionals, and other college (and high school) students can employ *Thirty Days to Better Nutrition* to improve their nutrition knowledge—as can anyone in search of reliable nutrition information.

Nutrition is a relatively new science. New developments seem to arise every day. Thus the nutrition information presented in this book may become outdated before the pages have a chance to wear out. At the present time, however, *Thirty Days to Better Nutrition* provides you with the most accurate, up-to-date, scientific facts on nutrition so that you can improve your diet, your health, and ultimately your overall well-being. You deserve it!

V.A.

DAY ONE
BALANCE THE BASICS

STEP 1: ATTITUDE

First, determine whether today is the right day for you to begin the Nutri-Plan by reading the following questions carefully and selecting your answers as honestly as possible.

Yes	No	Unsure	
☐	☐	☐	1. Do you feel motivated to improve your well-being?
☐	☐	☐	2. Are you willing to work at self-improvement for one entire month?
☐	☐	☐	3. Are you interested in learning the facts about diet and nutrition?
☐	☐	☐	4. Do you want to avoid diet foods and quick weight loss schemes?
☐	☐	☐	5. Are you anxious to begin now?
☐	☐	☐	6. Are you really in the mood for change?

If you were able to honestly answer Yes to at least five of the above questions, then today is probably a good day for you to start the Nutri-Plan. Ready, set, go! You have the necessary attitude.

If you answered No and/or Unsure to more than one of the above questions, then you may choose to wait until you are feeling more sure before beginning the Nutri-Plan. Instead, just read through Day One and answer the initial questions. If you still do not feel ready to devote yourself to the Nutri-Plan, then relax! There's always tomorrow, or next week, or even next month to begin improving yourself and your lifestyle. After all, you have many years of health-related habits and activities to consider, and many more years ahead in which to make any necessary alterations. And for many people, diet has become an added stress instead of a health-promoting (and fun!) part of life.

In order for you to be able to make successful changes in your lifestyle—to alter your diet and increase your knowledge of nutrition and health—it is extremely important for you to want to do so. A willing attitude with the motivation necessary for improving health and well-being is the first step—and the psychological foundation—for you to begin the Nutri-Plan.

STEP 2: A LOOK AT LIFESTYLE

How healthy do you think your lifestyle is? It is quite common to live from day to day—working, raising a family, socializing—without ever stopping to think about improving the quality of your present (and possibly the length of your future) life, simply by adopting a healthier lifestyle. You probably know how optimistic you can feel about life itself when you feel healthy. Yet, do you feel this healthy optimism every day, or only on occasion? Evaluate your own health-related habits by reading the following statements and selecting those answers which typically suit you:

Yes	No	
☐	☐	1) I get seven to eight hours of sleep every night.
☐	☐	2) I do not smoke cigarettes.
☐	☐	3) I drink alcohol in moderate amounts.
☐	☐	4) I exercise every day.
☐	☐	5) I eat breakfast every morning.
☐	☐	6) I eat regular meals every day.
☐	☐	7) I am at my desired weight.

If you were able to honestly answer Yes to all of the above statements, you probably have quite a healthy lifestyle. Congratulations!

However, if like most Americans, you had to answer No to more than one of the above statements, you may be cutting down your total lifespan! According to the results of a well-known study (conducted at UCLA in 1977 by Bellac and

Breslow), men who adhere to six out of these seven "health habits" most of the time can expect to live 11 years longer (women can expect to live seven years longer) than those who adhere to fewer than four!

And yet, almost all of the billions of dollars spent annually in the United States on health care go toward the treatment of sickness, rather than for the promotion of health. There are relatively few programs for early disease detection or health education. All too often, Americans do not simply die, but actually kill themselves! You can live a longer and healthier life, if you choose to.

STEP 3: A CLOSE LOOK AT DIET

Examine the role diet plays in your life by studying the following statements and selecting the answers which best suit you. Be honest with yourself!

Yes No
☐ ☐ 1) My diet is well balanced.
☐ ☐ 2) I avoid fad diets and quick weight loss schemes.
☐ ☐ 3) I try to help my family have well-balanced meals and snacks.
☐ ☐ 4) I talk about diet with friends and associates quite often.
☐ ☐ 5) I read articles and/or books on diet and nutrition.
☐ ☐ 6) I am aware of approximate calorie contents of many foods.
☐ ☐ 7) I am aware of general nutrient contents of many foods.
☐ ☐ 8) Diet is an integral component of my lifestyle: I am what I eat.

If you were able to honestly answer Yes to at least five of the above statements, then diet does seem to play an important role in your life. And because diet is so important to you, understanding how to balance your diet properly is essential!

If you found yourself selecting many No answers for the above statements, you may want to stop and ask yourself just how important you think diet is—for your physical self, intellectual self, and emotional self. If you think that your diet is important to you, then it is essential that you know how to balance it properly!

STEP 4: A CLOSER LOOK AT DIET

With 10,000 to 15,000 different items available in the typical supermarket, it may seem like a confusing chore for you to select foods wisely in order to eat a balanced diet. Actually, a well-balanced (and tasty!) diet can be achieved very simply, with a little nutrition know-how ...

Nutrients are the chemical substances we obtain from foods. Nutrients are essential for:

- the growth, upkeep, and repair of body tissues.
- the regulation of body processes.
- energy for the body.

No single food contains the 55 or so nutrients that the body requires in amounts adequate for proper growth and health. However, all of the nutrients we need can be provided by foods. A well-balanced diet contains the proper array of nutrients, and since foods vary in the kinds and amounts of nutrients they provide, it is important to include a variety of foods in the diet each day.

How varied is *your* diet? In each statement below, fill in the numbers which most closely approximate your typical dietary habits.

1) I usually include _____ servings of whole grain or enriched cereal, bread, pasta, rice, or other grains every *day*.

2) I usually include _____ servings of oranges, grapefruit, tomatoes or their juices every *day*.

3) I usually include _____ servings of dark green leafy vegetables (collard greens, kale, mustard greens, spinach, Swiss chard, etc) or bright yellow fruits or vegetables (apricots, carrots, pumpkin, squash, etc) each *week*.

4) I usually include _____ servings of other fruits and vegetables every *day*.

5) I usually drink _____ cups of milk every *day*; I eat _____ servings of cheese *daily*; I eat _____ cups of yogurt each *day*.

6) I usually include _____ servings of meat, poultry, or fish every *day*; I eat _____ eggs each *week*; I eat _____ cups of dried beans or peas (blackeyed peas, cowpeas, lentils, navy beans, pea beans, soybeans, etc) each *week*.

7) I usually include _____ servings of one or more of the following each *week*: cake, candy, cookies, donuts, jams, jellies, gum, pastries, pies, soft drinks, sugar, syrups.

8) I usually include _____ servings of one or more of the following each *week*: chips, crackers, dips, dried or smoked meats, salted nuts, pickles, pretzels, soups.

9) I usually drink _____ alcoholic beverages each *week*.

10) I usually drink _____ cups of coffee, tea, or cocoa every *day*.

11) I usually eat at fast food restaurants (fried chicken or seafood, hamburgers, hot dogs, pizza, tacos, etc) _____ times every *week*.

12) I consider my own diet to be:
   ☐ well-balanced and varied.
   ☐ unbalanced.
   ☐ repetitive.
   ☐ generally poor.

Remember, a well-balanced diet contains a variety of foods in order to include the proper array of nutrients.

Nutrients are separated according to their chemical compositions into six categories:

• Protein
• Carbohydrate
• Fat
• Vitamins
• Minerals
• Water

Nutritionists have incorporated both the bodily needs of individuals and the nutritive values of foods into:

The Basic Food Groups

The five groups separate foods in accordance with the similarities of their individual nutrient contents. Each group includes a variety of different foods with similar nutrient compositions. You can ensure an adequate intake of the needed nutrients by including in your diet the recommended number of daily servings of various foods from four of the basic food groups:

• Fruit and Vegetable Group
• Grain Group
• Milk and Cheese Group
• Meat and Alternates Group

The Others Group includes those foods for which the overall nutrient content is outweighed by the caloric content. These foods typically contain appreciable amounts of one or more of the following:

• Fat
• Sugar
• Salt
• Alcohol

Your body does not require a specific number of servings from the Others Group. If you choose to include some of these foods, serving sizes should be moderate.

Nutritional supplements are usually unnecessary for the normal, healthy individual who has a well-balanced diet including a variety of foods.

Is your diet well balanced and varied? Compare your answers from the 12 statements on page 2 to the contents of a well-balanced diet as illustrated in the chart below.

In order to approximate the well-balanced diet illustrated below, your answers from the twelve statements should be as follows: 1) four or more; 2) one or more; 3) three or more; 4) three or more; 5) Total = two (adult), three (child), four (teen); 6) two; three or less; one or more; 7–11) The lower

Basic Food Group	No. Servings Per Day	Serving Size	Food Sources
Fruit and Vegetable	4	½ cup juice	Citrus fruit or juice daily
		1 cup raw or ½ cup cooked	Dark green leafy vegetable or bright yellow fruit/vegetable 3–4 times per week Starchy vegetables are included in Grain group
Grain	4	1 slice ½–¾ cup ½ cup ⅓–½ cup	Bread—whole grain or enriched Cereal—cooked, dry, flours, grains Pasta—macaroni, noodles, spaghetti Starchy vegetables—corn, lima beans, peas, potato, pumpkin, winter squash
Milk and Cheese	2 (adult) 3 (child) 4 (teen)	1 cup 1½ oz 1 cup	Milk—buttermilk, skim, whole Cheese (calcium contents are higher in harder varieties) Yogurt
Meat and Alternates	2	2 oz cooked 2 1½ oz 1 cup 4 tbsp 1 cup	Meat, poultry, fish Eggs Cheese Cottage cheese Peanut butter, nuts Dried beans or peas
Others	—		Sweets—candy, cake, cookies, donuts, gum, jams, jellies, pastries, pies, soft drinks, sugars, syrups Alcoholic beverages—beer, wine, liquors, liqueurs, cordials Fats—butter, margarine, oils, salad dressings, shortening, bacon, cream, olives, avocado

the numbers, the better; 12) Your answer may spur you to read on!

Again, a well-balanced diet includes a varied intake of foods selected from the basic food groups, with the proper array of nutrients in the amounts necessary for health and well-being. Simple, yet so important!

STEP 5: 24-HOUR DIET RECALL

Once you have taken a general look at your dietary intake, you may want to take a close look at a specific day's intake. This may help you to better visualize your own personal food habits. Although one day is not representative of every day's food intake, an overview may enlighten you concerning some necessary dietary changes.

On the 24-Hour Diet Recall chart below, record everything that you have had to eat or drink during the past 24 hours. Include all meals, snacks, nibblings, beverages, coffee, etc. Record the approximate amount of each food eaten, as you remember it. Start with your most recent meal or snack and think back over the past 24 hours, recording as you recall each item. Use the Sample Diet Recall as a guide.

Sample Diet Recall

Day and Time	Food and Amount

Monday 9:00 am	Coffee - 1 cup
	    with creamer - 1 tbsp
	    and sugar - 2 tsp
	
	Toast, white - 1 slice
	    with butter - 1 pat
	    and jam, strawberry - 1 tbsp

Monday 7:30 am	Coffee - 1 cup
	    with creamer - 1 tbsp
	    and sugar - 2 tsp

Sunday 11:30 pm	Orange soda - 12 oz can Crackers, saltines - 10 or 12 with peanut butter - 3 tbsp
Sunday 9:00–10:00 pm	Chocolate candies - 2 handfuls Peanuts, dry roasted - 2 handfuls

Sunday 6:45 pm	French toast:
	    bread, white - 4 slices
	    egg (batter) - 2 to 3
	    butter - 3 tbsp
	    syrup - 4 tbsp
	Milk, whole - 1 cup

Sunday 2:00 pm	Martini - 4 oz
	Roast beef - 5 to 6 oz
	French fried potatoes - 12 to 15
	Green beans - ½ cup
	    with butter - 1 pat
	Roll, plain - 1 small
	    with butter - 1 pat
	Apple pie, homemade - average slice

Sunday 1:00–2:00 pm	Nibbled on: roast beef
	        French fried potatoes
	        Nuts
	        Onion dip 'n chips

Sunday 10:00 am	Coffee, black - 2 cups Donuts (chocolate, jelly) - 2

24-Hour Diet Recall

Day and Time	Food and Amount

Now, compare your food intake with the recommended servings from the basic food groups.

- Are you missing out entirely on any food group(s)?
- Are you low in the number of servings from any particular group(s)?
- How many servings have you included from the Others Group during the past 24 hours?

Every day is different, and you may feel that your 24-hour diet recall is not a fair representation of a typical day's food intake. Yet, you can definitely see that there is room for dietary improvement. Here's your chance to begin!

STEP 6: DAY ONE PLAN

Starting right now, record everything that you eat and drink in the Nutri-Plan diet diary (Appendix A). Make enough copies of this chart to provide you with ample space for recording 17 days of food intake and associated events. Be sure to record each food and beverage immediately after consumption, for two reasons:

- If you wait until the end of each day to recall your food intake, you may forget some of what you ate or drank (eg, nibblings, snacks, coffee).
- The knowledge that you must record every item which enters your mouth may help you to resist impulsive indulgences.

Make your food descriptions quite specific as details can provide you with vivid recollections of your intakes for later use. Note that approximate intake amounts are also to be recorded. It is important for you to become aware not only of what you eat, but also of how much. Also record the length of time you spend in eating each meal or snack. You may want to begin to note whether you relax and enjoy your food, or if you tend to hurriedly wolf it down.

Try to determine how hungry you are every time you eat, and rate your hunger as:

PH - Physically hungry (stomach feels empty, "growls," etc)
EH - Emotionally hungry (desire food to appease tension, stress, anger, boredom, fatigue, etc)
OH - Outside/environmentally hungry (sight or smell of food causes eating, social pressures to eat, eating due to time such as "lunch hour," etc)

Record also any comments or personal feelings you may have concerning your food intake and your hunger. Be honest with yourself. Failure to record food intake or to report true feelings will prevent you from learning about your personal food habits. You will only be hurting yourself!

If utilized properly, your Nutri-Plan diet diary can eventually do the following:

- reveal to you the true quantities of your intake of different foods and beverages.
- help you to identify those foods and beverages you may need to decrease in your diet.
- help you to identify those items you may need to increase in your diet.
- indicate the need for alterations in your typical eating speeds.
- reveal to you certain personal snacking or nibbling habits you may be unaware of.
- help you to differentiate between your physical need for food and various emotional or environmental influences on your eating behaviors.
- provide you with increased insight into your own individual eating habits.
- serve as the basis for making changes in your diet, while providing you with the means for observing these changes.

DAY TWO

PROTEIN POWER

STEP 1: SEPARATING FACT FROM FANCY

The 55 or so nutrients essential for proper body growth and function are separated into six categories.

- Protein
- Carbohydrate
- Fat
- Vitamins
- Minerals
- Water

No single category can provide the body with all that is required in order to build new tissue and to work smoothly and efficiently. Day by day, as the month progresses, you will learn some of the basics about each of these six important categories.

Today you can begin to examine protein. Try taking the following quiz in order to determine what you already know about protein. The answers are given throughout Day Two, and are also listed under Step 5.

Indicate if the following statements are True or False:

True False

☐ ☐ 1) Meat is our only source of high quality protein.

☐ ☐ 2) Protein is the second most abundant substance in our bodies.

☐ ☐ 3) High quality protein contains adequate amounts of all of the essential amino acids.

☐ ☐ 4) There are only five essential amino acids which must be obtained through diet.

☐ ☐ 5) Plant proteins do not contain adequate amino acids, so cannot serve as a valid protein source.

☐ ☐ 6) Protein undernutrition is fairly common in America today.

☐ ☐ 7) Athletes need much larger quantities of dietary protein than are normally required.

☐ ☐ 8) A high-protein diet has been shown to be an effective method for permanent weight loss.

Protein is required for life itself, and is found in the cells of all plants and animals. Plants make their own special protein while animals, in most cases, must rely on ingested sources of protein. To most Americans, "protein" means "meat," but high quality protein is also provided by poultry, fish, eggs, cheese, milk, yogurt, and specific plant combinations.

Next to water, protein is the most abundant substance present in our bodies, contributing around twenty percent of total body weight. Protein helps to form hair, nails, skin, bones, and muscles. Protein is essential to oxygen transport in the bloodstream, blood sugar regulation, clotting mechanisms, and systems for protection against infection. Protein also forms enzymes which speed up body processes, and the hormones which regulate these body processes.

STEP 2: BEADS AND NECKLACES

Protein is composed of 22 building blocks known as "amino acids," linked together in various combinations like the beads on a necklace. The number of possible combinations is almost infinite, and tens of thousands of the same amino acids might even be repeated in a single protein. Thus, amino acids (beads) form a wide variety of patterns (necklaces):

During digestion, the amino acid chains in protein foods are broken, and later rearranged to form body proteins. In order to build body protein efficiently, a well-balanced mixture of amino acids must be present. If the amino acids available are not properly balanced (ie, certain amino acids are low or missing), protein cannot be built and the amino acids are wasted. It is as if certain beads are missing from a necklace so that a desired pattern cannot be formed, and therefore the necklace cannot be strung:

o⃞o⃞o⃞o⃞o⃞o DESIRED NECKLACE / AMINO ACID PATTERN

-o-o-   ⃞ ⃞ ⃞ ⃞   AVAILABLE BEADS/AMINO ACIDS

o⃞o⃞   INCOMPLETE PATTERN WITH

   ⃞ ⃞   "WASTED" BEADS / AMINO ACIDS

Some of the 22 necessary amino acids can be manufactured by our bodies, but 9 cannot be synthesized at a rate sufficient to meet our needs. These 9 so-called "essential" amino acids must be provided by foods, while the 13 "nonessential" amino acids can be manufactured within the body from ingested dietary protein.

A high quality protein provides all of the essential amino acids in those proportions required by the body. Because the composition of the animal body is similar to that of the human body, the amino acid balance of animal foods (meat, poultry, fish, eggs, cheese, milk, yogurt) is of higher quality than that of plant foods. Plant proteins do not contain the proper assortment of amino acids in the amounts sufficient to support bodily growth. Therefore, plant foods should be combined with animal foods in order to improve the quality of the available protein. Also, so-called "complementary" plant foods can contribute high quality protein to the diet:

PLANT FOOD #1:   PLANT FOOD #2:
       Complementary with   HIGH QUALITY PROTEIN MEAL:

Choose the two plant foods with complementary proteins from the selections below, in order to form the following high quality protein:

PLANT FOOD #1:   PLANT FOOD #2:   PLANT FOOD #3:   PLANT FOOD #4:

If you chose Plant Food #2 and Plant Food #3, you were then able to form the high quality protein illustrated above.

STEP 3: COMPLEMENTARY FOOD SELECTION

In the real plant kingdom, complementary pairing is as follows:

Corn	↔	Beans, Peanuts, Soy
Rice	↔	Beans, Peanuts
Wheat	↔	All Legumes
Oats	↔	Peanuts
Rye	↔	Soy
Sesame	↔	Garbanzos, Soy

And remember that whenever any of the plant foods are combined with animal foods, the resulting protein is of high quality.

Using the pairing given above, select the food combinations which are complementary, and therefore provide high quality protein. Note that in several cases there may be more than one complementary food pairing, so that there may also be more than one correct answer.

1) Whole wheat cereal and _____.
   a) milk   b) banana   c) raisins
2) Corn tortillas and _____.
   a) refried beans   b) cheddar cheese
   c) green peppers
3) Brown rice and _____.
   a) stir-fried mushrooms   b) peanuts
   c) tomato sauce
4) Oatmeal bread and _____.
   a) peanut butter   b) margarine
   c) Swiss cheese
5) Sesame seeds and _____.
   a) brown rice   b) cheese sauce over broccoli
   c) garbanzos on a tossed salad

Your answers should have been as follows: 1) a
2) a,b   3) b   4) a,c   5)b,c

In order to use complementary foods in your own cooking and menu planning, simply cut out the handy chart given below. You might want to

attach the chart to your refrigerator or a kitchen cabinet to allow for easy referral.

STEP 4: HOW MUCH?

Our bodies need protein of high quality. What about quantity?

Protein undernutrition is rare in America today. Most of us, in fact, consume two to three times more protein than our bodies actually need. A regular, continuous supply of dietary protein is desirable because the body has little protein reserve. If more protein is consumed than is needed, however, the excess will be used for energy, if necessary, or stored as body fat.

Our need for protein is heightened when we are building new tissue at a rapid rate (eg, during infancy and pregnancy), and following tissue destruction (eg, after hemorrhage, burns, or surgery). Contrary to popular belief, athletes require little, if any, extra protein in their diets. From the standpoint of energy production, only 5% to 15% of total energy in the well-nourished individual is from protein breakdown. Thus, the protein used for muscle power is actually quite small so that, except for the small amount of protein required by developing muscles during conditioning, protein requirements are not increased for the athlete. And since most of us obtain more protein than we need anyway, it is unlikely that the well-nourished athlete will require extra or supplemental protein.

Use the following chart to assist you in determining the approximate number of grams of protein you should obtain each day in order to meet your own needs. In order to convert your weight in pounds into kilograms (kg) simply divide by 2.2. The recommended amounts were determined in 1980 by the National Research Council's Food and Nutrition Board, US National Academy of Sciences.

Individual Status*	Recommended Daily Intake of Protein in Grams
Infancy–6 months	2.4–2.0/kg body weight
6 months–1 year	2.0/kg body weight
Childhood–adolescence	2.0–0.8/kg body weight
Adulthood	0.8/kg body weight
Pregnancy	0.8/kg body weight + 10 grams
Lactation	0.8/kg body weight + 20 grams

*Note that protein requirements decline gradually with age.

STEP 5: HIGH PROTEIN DIET

Dieters are often encouraged by the initial rapid loss of weight achieved on a high-protein diet. Results, however, are usually only temporary. A

Complementary Foods—Easy Reference Chart	
Plant Foods ◄────►	Animal Foods (meat, poultry, fish, eggs, cheese, milk, yogurt)
Legumes (dried beans and peas) ◄────►	Grains (barley, buckwheat, corn, oats, millet, rice, rye, wheat)
Legumes ◄────►	Nuts
Legumes ◄────►	Seeds

high intake of protein and/or a low intake of carbohydrate results in loss of body fluids. Since body fluid weighs as much as body fat, weight loss does result—but it is loss of fluid, not loss of undesirable body fat, which accounts for most of this weight loss! A high-protein diet is not more effective than a low-calorie diet in achieving loss of body fat. It is the total number of calories consumed, rather than the kind of food eaten, that is essential in achieving permanent weight loss. And it is changes in eating behaviors—permanent changes—which lead to successful weight loss and effective maintenance of the loss. (On Days Nine and Sixteen through Twenty-three you will learn more about effective weight control and can begin to incorporate the concepts into your own lifestyle.)

Possible harmful side effects from an exclusively high-protein regime range from dizziness and fatigue to dehydration, kidney disorders, and even death. Remember the once popular, now banned "liquid protein" diets? These were accountable for around 50 deaths in United States!

From the list below, select the diet which you believe would be most effective in achieving safe, permanent weight loss:

_____ (a) High-protein diet
_____ (b) Low-carbohydrate diet
_____ (c) Complementary plant food diet
_____ (d) Starvation diet
_____ (e) Water only diet
_____ (f) Low-calorie, well-balanced diet

The best diet for permanent success is selection (f), which is not as dull as you may think. It is obvious now, from the information given on Day One, that a well-balanced diet is most desirable from the standpoint of good health, and an easy method for you to keep track of calories as well as nutrients will be explained in upcoming Days. In fact, by Day Thirty the well-balanced, calorie-controlled way of eating may be an integral part of your lifestyle!

The answers to the quiz from Step 1 are given throughout Day Two. Use the following key to recheck your answers:

1. False   2. True   3. True   4. False
5. False   6. False   7. False   8. False

STEP 6: YOUR PROTEIN POWER

Use your Nutri-Plan diet diary (Appendix A) and a chart which lists the protein contents of common foods (see Recommended References) in order to determine whether you obtained the recommended amount of protein on Day One. In the chart on page 11, list all foods eaten on Day One and the amounts. Then calculate the grams of protein for each item using the information provided in the nutrient values chart and total your protein intake for Day One. (Actual protein values may be higher when plant foods are consumed with animal foods and when complementary plant foods are eaten.)

Now compare this total to your individual recommended daily intake, as determined in Step 4.

Did you consume twice as much protein as required? Three times as much? Or did you fail to obtain enough protein to meet your needs for the day? Note that this is only an estimate, since protein absorption varies depending on the food itself, its preparation, the individual consumer, and other factors.

STEP 7: DAY TWO PLAN

Continue to record everything you eat and drink in your Nutri-Plan diet diary. Be sure to record each food and beverage immediately after consumption. Be specific in describing foods and amounts, and continue to observe length of meal times and types of hunger. Record any comments and feelings you may have concerning your intake and your hunger. Remember to be honest and you may begin to gain valuable insight into your own personal food habits.

For Day Two, begin to observe your protein intake. Use a nutrient value chart to determine the protein value for each food and beverage you plan to consume. Try to include the amount of protein appropriate for your own needs, as determined in Step 4. See how close you can approximate your recommended daily intake. If you see by bedtime that your protein intake is too low, select a high quality protein snack (eg, peanut butter on wheat bread or cheese and crackers). If you notice that by dinnertime your protein intake is already excessive, keep additional protein servings to a minimum (eg, instead of six ounces of chicken, eat only three ounces or stretch two ounces by making chicken salad or a casserole). Total your protein intake (in grams) for Day Two and compare to your individual recommended daily intake.

Day One

Food and Amount	Protein (g)

Total Protein:_____ g
Your Individual Recommended Dietary Intake:
_____ g

DAY THREE

CARBO-HABITS

STEP 1: IDENTIFYING CARBOHYDRATES

Most of the world's people obtain about 70% of their total caloric intake as carbohydrate, while Americans receive only around 45% of their total calories in this form. Americans tend to include the lesser amount of carbohydrate in their diets because:

- Most consume a large amount of protein, often more than twice the recommended amounts (see Day Two).
- Many mistakenly believe that all carbohydrate foods are high in calories and low in nutritional value.
- Many consider carbohydrate foods to be unnecessary expenses, even though they are actually quite economical to produce in abundance.

Carbohydrate can prove to be an economical, nutritional, and psychological boon to your lifestyle: with a little carbohydrate know-how, you can decrease your food bills, control your weight, and balance your diet!

Carbohydrates in our diets come in two major forms:

- Sugars
- Starches

The simple sugars (monosaccharides) are the building blocks for most common carbohydrates. They double up to form double sugars (disaccharides) and connect in chains of three or more to form the more complex starches (polysaccharides). In order for the body to be able to use them, carbohydrates must be broken down during digestion into simple sugars. The carbohydrate material which the human body is unable to fully break down is known as fiber. Although it does not provide us with either energy or nutrients, fiber is an important dietary constituent. Fiber is essential to the proper function of the gastrointestinal system, assisting in digestion, elimination, and in the prevention of certain diseases. (Days Eleven and Twelve discuss fiber in more detail.)

In order to identify carbohydrates, some familiarity with the following terms is helpful:

Simple Sugars (Monosaccharides)	Glucose ("blood sugar") Fructose ("fruit sugar") Galactose
Double Sugars (Disaccharides)	Glucose + Fructose = Sucrose ("table sugar," brown sugar, honey, syrups) Glucose + Galactose = Lactose ("milk sugar") Glucose + Glucose = Maltose (malt products)
Starches (Polysaccharides)	Digestible ("starch," dextrins) Partially digestible Indigestible ("fiber," cellulose, hemi-cellulose, pectin)

Now examine the ingredient lists for the following hypothetical food products. Can you identify the kind(s) of carbohydrate in each item?

1)
YOGURT

"Ingredients: Milk, sugar, fruit..."
Carbohydrate(s)_____
a) lactose
b) sucrose
c) fructose
d) all of the above

2)
BEER

"Ingredients: Barley, malt, air bubbles..."
Carbohydrate(s)_____
a) starch
b) maltose
c) both of the above

3)
BREAD

"Ingredients: Wheat flour, honey, milk, bran..."
Carbohydrate(s)_____
a) starch
b) sucrose
c) lactose
d) all of the above

4)

CEREAL

"Ingredients: Whole rolled oats, dehydrated bananas, corn syrup..."

Carbohydrate(s)_____
a) starch
b) fructose
c) sucrose
d) all of the above

5)

ICE CREAM

"Ingredients: Cream, whole milk, honey, lemon..."

Carbohydrate(s)_____
a) lactose
b) sucrose
c) fructose
d) all of the above.

In each of the five examples, the last answer is the best choice.

STEP 2: NUTRIENTS IN SUGAR

The major function of carbohydrates is the provision of energy, but carbohydrate foods also serve as carriers of other important nutrients and fiber. The world's major carbohydrate sources are:

• cereal grains (barley, buckwheat, corn, millet, oats, rice, rye, wheat)
• potatoes
• fruits and vegetables
• dried beans and peas
• cassava (tapioca)
• sugar cane
• sugar beet

Many of our processed foods are also rich in carbohydrates, including such products as:

• breads and other baked goods
• pastas
• dried fruits
• jams and jellies
• molasses, honey, syrups
• desserts

Many carbohydrate foods contain a combination of sugars and starches, as illustrated by the hypothetical food products in Step 1. The most preferable carbohydrate foods, however, also contain a combination of essential nutrients and/or fiber.

From sugar cane and sugar beet we derive refined "table sugar" (sucrose), which is basically pure carbohydrate. Table sugar provides calories without any accompanying nutrients. Brown sugar, "raw sugar" (which is actually refined), and honey provide, in addition to carbohydrate, only trace amounts of a few nutrients. Molasses does

contain an appreciable amount of iron.

Try to guess the nutrient equivalencies for the following foods:

1) In order to obtain the amount of calcium provided by one cup of skim milk, you would have to consume _____ tablespoons of honey.
   a) 2–3   b) 10   c) 296

2) In order to obtain the amount of iron found in a pint of clams you would have to eat _____ tablespoons of brown sugar.
   a) 3   b) 13   c) 113

3) In order to obtain the amount of potassium provided by an orange, you would have to consume _____ tablespoons of honey.
   a) 2   b) 12   c) 24

In each case the answer is c), the largest amount given. And when you consider the fact that one cup of skim milk provides fewer than 90 calories, while 296 tablespoons of honey is equivalent to almost 19,000 calories, the point becomes even clearer: refined sugar provides carbohydrate and calories with little, if any, accompanying nutrients.

STEP 3: HOW MUCH SUGAR?

Americans now consume over 100 pounds of refined sugars per person each year! This is partially due to our increased consumption of many processed foods with high sugar contents, in particular:

• Soft drinks
• Bakery items
• Candy
• Presweetened cereals
• Sweet desserts

These foods provide carbohydrates and calories, but usually contain negligible amounts of other nutrients and fiber. Compare the nutrients and calories provided by an average daily intake of table sugar with the nutrients and calories found in comparable amounts of several other carbohydrate foods (see top of page 15).

Do you see the nutritional differences?

STEP 4: IT ALL ADDS UP

Sugar is known to be detrimental to dental health (more on this painful subject on Day Fifteen), yet, we continue to enjoy sugary foods. Highly sweetened foods can contribute a considerable number of calories to the diet without ad-

	1 CUP SUGAR	1 CUP WHOLE WHEAT FLOUR	1 LARGE POTATO	1 EAR CORN	1 CUP BAKED BEANS
Calories:	770	400	145	130	224
Vitamins:	trace	good source B-vitamins	good source vitamin C	good source vitamin A	good source B-vitamins
Iron:	.2 mg	4.0	1.1 mg	1.3 mg	5.1 mg
Fiber:	none	good source	good source with skin	good source	good source

ding many nutrients. Sweets often taste good, so we tend to overeat them. Thus, when combined with the large number of processed foods with added sugar which now comprise the typical American diet, the daily number of sweet calories we consume can easily add up...and up!

Compare the caloric contents of some carbohydrate foods which are low in sugar with the calories in some of our popular sweets:

Wheat bread, 1 slice	70 calories
Banana bread, 1/12 loaf	170 calories
Donut, plain	150 calories
Danish pastry	270 calories
Pancake, 3" diameter	80 calories
Pancake with syrup, 3 tbsp	230 calories
Pumpkin, mashed	80 calories
Pumpkin pie, 1/8 of 9" pie	240 calories
Rice, 1/2 cup	90 calories
Rice pudding, 1/2 cup	190 calories
Rice pudding, 1/2 cup with vanilla ice cream, 1/2 cup	340 calories

Note that some of the more caloric items above contain a considerable amount of fat which also contributes to total calories. (More on fats on Day Four).

Actually, much of the increase in sugar consumption during the past 40 years is due to the expanded use of corn sweeteners in processing. Corn sweeteners are added to a wide variety of processed foods, including many products which we do not even think of as sweet. Careful label examination will reveal the presence of corn sweeteners in such unsuspected items as:

- Noodle mixes
- Salad dressings
- Catsup
- Soups
- Frozen dinners
- Chips and snack foods

How much sugar do you think you consume in a typical day? Over an entire year? Nowhere near one hundred pounds you say? Keep this in mind—you may shock yourself on Day Fifteen.

STEP 5: ON STARCH

Our bodies do not require any refined sugar. We can obtain all of the energy we need, plus various nutrients and fiber, from the natural sugars and starch available in such carbohydrate foods as milk, fruits, vegetables, whole grain breads, and cereals.

Take a look at the chart on page 16 which lists some common starchy foods. Note that all are rich in fiber content, relatively low in calories, and offer considerable amounts of several important vitamins and minerals.

STEP 6: STARCH VS SUGAR

Do you tend to avoid starchy foods? Do you actually eat more sugar than you realize? The next chart can assist you in observing your own carbo-habits for one day. See sample chart on page 16.

First, look at Day Two of your Nutri-Plan diet diary and list in Column A all foods consumed which are listed in the chart given in Step 5. Next, list in Column B all foods and beverages consumed on Day Two which contain a significant amount of refined sugars (eg, soft drinks, bakery items, candy, presweetened cereals, sweet desserts, jams and jellies, honey, molasses, syrups, etc). Note that some foods contain appreciable amounts of both starch and sugar, so can be included in both columns. Total the numbers of starchy food servings (Column A), and compare the result to the total number of sugar-rich food servings (Column B). What are *your* carbo-habits?

Food	Fiber	Calories/Cup	Notable Nutrients
Cereal Grains:	Good Source		
Barley	"	696	Potassium, B-Vitamins
Buckwheat*	"	340	Potassium
Corn	"	137	Potassium, Vitamin A
Millet	"	760	Potassium, B-Vitamins
Oats	"	312	Potassium, B-Vitamins
Rice (Brown)	"	666	Potassium, B-Vitamins
Rye	"	364	B-Vitamins
Wheat*	"	400	Potassium, B-Vitamins
Legumes:			
Dried Beans	"	224	Iron, Potassium, B-Vitamins
Dried Peas	"	230	Iron, Potassium, B-Vitamins
Lentils	"	212	Iron, Potassium, B-Vitamins
Soybeans	"	234	Iron, Potassium, B-Vitamins
Starchy Vegetables			
Lima Beans	"	189	Calcium, Iron, Potassium, Vitamin A, B-Vitamins
Parsnips	"	139	Potassium, B-Vitamins
Peas	"	114	Potassium, Vitamin A, B-Vitamins
Potato	"	145	Iron, Potassium, Vitamin C
Sweet Potato	"	161	Potassium, Vitamin A

*Cracked Wheat = Bulgur
 Cracked Buckwheat = Kasha

STEP 7: DAY THREE PLAN

Continue to record everything you eat and drink in your Nutri-Plan diet diary. For Day Three, continue to be aware of your protein intake and try to approximate your personal needs. Also, begin to observe your carbohydrate intake. Try to include foods in your diet which are rich in starch and minimize your intake of foods high in refined sugar. Then, at the end of Day Three, complete another chart like the one in Step 6 and compare the totals to the totals from Day Two. Did you notice any improvement over Day Two? Could it be simply a matter of awareness?

SAMPLE CHART

Column A: Starchy Foods and Amounts	No. of Servings	Column B: Sugar-Rich Foods and Amounts	No. of Servings
Oatmeal, ¾ cup	1	Sugar (in coffee), 2 tsp.	2
Wheat bread, 2 slices	2	Donut	1
Baked potato, med.	1	Jam, 2 tsp.	2
Corn on the cob, 1 ear	1	Lemonade, 1 cup	1
Rice pudding, ½ cup	1	Cranberry sauce, ¼ cup	1
Wheat crackers, 4	1	Rice pudding, ½ cup	1
		Ice cream, ½ cup	1
		Lifesavers, 2	2
Total No. of Servings	7	Total No. of Servings	11

Day Two

Starchy Foods and Amounts	No. of Servings	Sugar-Rich Foods and Amounts	No. of Servings
Total No. of Servings		Total No. of Servings	

DAY FOUR

FAT FACTS

STEP 1: FAT CALORIES

For many years, Americans considered all protein foods to be "good," and all carbohydrate foods to be "bad." From the information provided in Day Two and Day Three, you are now able to discount this misconception. Food fat, however, should not be ignored. In fact, dietary fat is thought to be a contributing factor in the development of certain diseases. There is much to learn on the subject of food fat; this information will not only help you to improve your dietary status, but may aid in the prevention of disease as well.

First, try to match each nutrient listed below with the approximate number of calories it provides. Answers are given immediately following.

Nutrient	Calories per gram (or ounce)
____ Protein	a) 0 (or 0)
____ Carbohydrate	b) 4 (or 115)
____ Fat	c) 100 (or 2800)
____ Vitamins	d) 10 (or 280)
____ Minerals	e) 1 (or 25)
____ Water	f) 9 (or 250)

It may surprise you to learn that fat actually provides more than twice as many calories per gram (or ounce) as both protein and carbohydrate. The latter two nutrients each provide approximately four calories per gram (or 115 calories per ounce), while fat provides a whopping nine calories per gram (or 250 calories per ounce)! One tablespoon of vegetable oil provides you with around 120 calories, which makes vegetable oil the most concentrated source of calories found in your kitchen.

Vitamins, minerals, and water are not energy-providing nutrients, and they do not supply any calories at all.

STEP 2: WHERE ARE THE FAT CALORIES FOUND?

Since Americans are amongst the world's greatest consumers of protein, it is surprising to learn that protein provides only about 15% of our total caloric intake—and most of us actually require about half this amount.

The average American obtains approximately 40% of total caloric intake from fat. Why? How? Most foods thought to be rich in protein actually contain considerable amounts of fat, with protein supplying only a fraction of the total calories. So, by understanding the relatively small amount of protein our bodies require, and learning to recognize the actual amounts of protein found in our foods, we will then be able to identify food fat.

Examine the chart below to compare the caloric values of some "protein-rich" foods with the number of fat calories each provides.

Food and Amount	Total Calories	Fat Calories
Almonds - 10	60	50
Peanut butter - 1 tbsp	90	70
Peanuts - 10	110	80
Bologna - 1 oz	80	60
Bacon - 2 slices	90	70
Frankfurter - 1 small	130	100
Sausage - 1 link	170	140
Steak, flank - 6 oz	330	110
Steak, sirloin - 6 oz	660	490
Steak, t-bone - 10.4 oz	1400	1150
Tuna in water - 3 oz	120	8
Tuna in oil - 3 oz	150	60
Chicken, thigh - 3 oz	120	50
Egg - 1 medium	80	50
Cheese, cottage - ½ cup	110	40
Cheese, cheddar - 1 oz	110	80
Cheese, cream - 1 oz	120	100
Milk, skim - 1 cup	90	2
Milk, whole - 1 cup	160	80
Ice cream - 1 cup	260	180

Remember that fat yields nine calories per gram (or 250 per ounce), so serves as a concentrated calorie source. The chart above clearly illustrates how some seemingly protein-rich, low-calorie foods actually provide concentrated amounts of calories in the form of fat. These fat calories can add up... and up!

STEP 3: VISIBLE OR HIDDEN?

Control over fat intake has two main principles:

- the AMOUNT of fat
- the KIND of fat

It is quite easy for us to misjudge and underestimate the amount of fat found in a food. This is because fat is a concentrated source of energy, and what appears to be only a "dab" of fat may turn out to be worth over a hundred calories!

Food fat may be visible, or it can be hidden. Try to determine whether each of the foods listed below contains any fat. If so, indicate by (✔) whether the fat is visible or hidden. The first one has been done for you. Answers are given below.

Food	Contains Fat (✔)	Visible Fat (✔)	or	Hidden Fat (✔)
1. Butter	✔	✔		
2. Salad dressing				
3. French fries				
4. Cola				
5. Oatmeal				
6. Peanut butter				
7. Avocado				
8. Egg, hard-cooked				
9. Cheese, cheddar				
10. Yogurt, plain				
11. Liver, broiled				
12. Turkey, without skin				
13. Donut, plain				
14. Milk chocolate bar				
15. Olive				

In the chart above, only numbers 4 and 5 (cola and oatmeal) do not contain fat. Numbers 1, 2, and 3 (butter, salad dressing, and French fries) contain visible fat: we can see the fat present in butter, margarine, shortening, cooking and salad oils; it is also possible to observe some of the fatty, greasy fat found in fried foods.

The rest of the foods listed above, numbers 6 through 15, contain hidden fat: we are unable to see many of the particles of fat present in meats, poultry, fish, eggs, nuts, and whole or low-fat milk, cheese and yogurt. Many processed foods (such as pastries, pies, cakes, cookies, ice cream, sauces, gravies, luncheon meats, chips, etc) also contain considerable amounts of hidden fat. The chart below illustrates how certain seemingly innocent foods are actually high in calories due to their hidden fat contents.

Food and Amount	Total Calories	Fat Calories
Avocado, med. size, ½	140	130
Chocolate candy, sm. bar	150	80
Olives, 10 large	45	45
Fish sticks, 2	100	50
Omelet, 2 eggs	220	150
Walnuts, chopped, 1 tbsp	50	40
Yogurt, whole milk, 1 cup	150	70
Soup, cream of mushroom, 1 cup	220	130
Potato, mashed, ½ cup	90	35
Donut, raised	180	100
Cookie, sandwich	50	20
French fries, 10	170	60

STEP 4: KINDS OF FAT

Fat is an integral dietary component. Food fat provides us with the following:

- calories for body energy
- palatability to enhance the flavor of food
- satiety value to aid the feeling of "fullness"
- fatty acids essential for growth
- transport for certain vitamins

Evidence now exists, however, which links various diseases with high blood levels of certain types of fat. The kinds of fat included in the diet appear to influence the levels of fat in the blood. Thus, it becomes obvious that—in addition to the amount of fat—it is important to consider the kinds of fat included in the diet.

Although there is probably no need for most of us to memorize fat-related terms, a review of their definitions may shed some light on the general role of each—in your body, your diet, and in health or disease. Match each term listed below with the most appropriate definition and check your answers by referring to a medical dictionary (see Appendix C). Answers are given following Step 5.

Term	Definition
__ 1) Fatty acids	a) a general term for fats, including tri-glycerides, cholesterol, phospholipids, and dietary fats.
__ 2) Cholesterol	
__ 3) Saturated fats	
__ 4) Unsaturated fats	b) the building blocks of fats.
__ 5) Triglycerides	c) the most common form of lipid in the diet, and the usual storage form of fats in the body; these fats are rapidly absorbed from food and can be synthesized by the body from both sugar and alcohol.
__ 6) Lipid	
__ 7) HDL	
__ 8) Lipid profile	
__ 9) Hyperlipidemia	
__10) Atherosclerosis	

___11) Hydrogenation

d) a waxy, fat-like substance found in every animal cell which is manufactured by the liver, and is present in all foods of animal origin (especially egg yolk, organ meats, fatty meats, shrimp, butter, cream, whole milk, and whole milk cheeses).

e) fats that are usually hard at room temperature, found primarily in animal products (meat, eggs, lard, butter, cream, whole milk, and whole milk cheeses), and are abundant in solid and hydrogenated vegetable fats, coconut oil, palm oil, chocolate, some margarines, and shortening.

f) fats that are usually liquid at room temperature, and are abundant in plant seed oils (safflower, sunflower, corn, soybean, cottonseed, sesame, walnut, olive and peanut).

g) the chemical process used to convert unsaturated fats from liquid to semisolid form in order to make the product more saturated and thereby increase shelf life.

h) disease in which fatty plaques build on the artery walls, narrowing them and possibly resulting in heart attack or stroke.

i) condition characterized by an excess of fatty materials (cholesterol and/or tri-glycerides) in the blood.

j) laboratory test used to determine levels of fatty materials in the blood.

k) "high density lipoproteins"; elevated blood levels have been correlated with a decreased incidence of atherosclerosis.

STEP 5: FATS AND DISEASE

The average American diet contains 15% of the total calories as protein and 40% as fat. It has been recommended, however, that the amount of fat—and the amount of saturated fat in particular—should comprise only 30% of the total calories. This would leave 55% of the total calorie intake to be supplied by carbohydrate. And, as we learned on Day Three, wise selection of carbohydrate foods can provide us with low-calorie sources of a variety of important nutrients plus fiber.

Indicate (✓) which of the following diseases might possibly be related to dietary fat and/or cholesterol:

_____ 1) Heart disease
_____ 2) Atherosclerosis
_____ 3) Cancer of the colon
_____ 4) Cancer of the breast

The fat/cholesterol controversy will be discussed on Days Thirteen and Fourteen, but in the meantime you may want to keep in mind the following concepts:

- Heart disease is the number one killer in America today, accounting for more deaths than all other diseases combined.
- Most cultures which follow a diet rich in saturated fat and cholesterol demonstrate a high rate of atherosclerosis as well.
- A high-fat, high-cholesterol diet produces atherosclerosis in many species of laboratory animals.
- Recent studies indicate a possible relationship between a high-fat diet and cancer of the colon and breast.

*   *   *

The best definition for the terms listed in Step 4 are as follows:

1) b, 2) d, 3) e, 4) f, 5) c, 6) a, 7) k, 8) j, 9) i, 10) h, 11) g.

STEP 6: IDENTIFYING SATURATED FAT

Most sources of saturated fat are of animal origin and are usually solid at room temperature. Because they spoil less rapidly than most liquid fats, saturated fats are often included in processed foods.

Post the chart on page 23 on your refrigerator or kitchen cabinet. By being able to identify the presence of saturated fats in your foods, you can then control the amount in your daily diet.

STEP 7: FAT ON THE LABEL

Most of us consume diets which contain considerable amounts of processed foods. Therefore, in order that we may identify product ingredients, it is essential that we read food labels.

Take a few minutes to look at the labels on the foods listed below. You can use the products in your kitchen, or you may need to visit your local supermarket. Do any of the listed foods contain saturated fat? Use the supplemental list entitled "Sneaky Sources of Saturated Fats" on page 22 to assist you in identifying the possible sources of saturated fat. A sample has been done for you.

Food Labels to Examine	Saturated Fat Source
Donuts, packaged	"Shortening"
Margarine	
Nuts, roasted	
Non-dairy creamer	
Frozen dinner	
Cookies, packaged	
Crackers, cheese-flavored	
Soup, canned	
Peanut butter	

Remember, although fats are sometimes visible in foods, they are often hidden, and are added to many of our processed foods. It becomes your responsibility to be able to identify both the visible and the hidden fats in the foods you eat, and to control the amount and kinds of fat in your diet.

Sneaky Sources of Saturated Fats

Check food labels carefully for:

Coconut oil
Palm oil
Vegetable oil (type unidentified)
Hydrogenated oil
Partially hydrogenated oil
Shortening
Lard
Chicken fat (other meat fats)

STEP 8: FAT IN YOUR DIET

On a typical day, approximately how much saturated fat do you think you consume? Look at Day Three in your Nutri-Plan diet diary. On a separate sheet of paper, list all foods and beverages consumed. Underline the foods and beverages which contain fat; nutrient values charts may assist you (see Appendix C). Then, using the chart in Step 6, circle those items which probably contain saturated fat. Total all underlined items (fat). Total all circled items (saturated fat). Be sure to check food labels for ingredients whenever necessary. A sample chart is given here.

STEP 9: DAY FOUR PLAN

Continue to record everything you eat and drink in your Nutri-Plan diet diary. For Day Four, continue to be aware of both your protein and your carbohydrate intake. Try to approximate your needs, and to select foods wisely. Beware of excessive consumption of "meats and sweets," and try to include plenty of nutritious starch foods. Also, try to minimize your total fat intake. Be especially conscious of those foods which are high in saturated fat.

At the end of Day Four, complete another chart totaling the fats in your foods using the methods you utilized in Step 8. Can you see any improvement over Day Three (Step 8)? Are there fewer total underlined items (fat) on Day Four? Are there

Sample Chart
Day Three

Foods and Amounts
(AM) corn flakes - 1 cup
milk, whole - ½ cup
sugar - 1 tsp
toast - 1 sl
margarine - 1 tsp
coffee - 1 cup
creamer 1 tbsp
(Noon) sandwich: rye bread - 2 sl
bologna - 1 oz
cheddar cheese - 1 oz
mayonnaise - 1 tsp
mustard - 1 tsp
lettuce
cola - 12 oz can
chocolate chip cookies - 2 lg
(Snack) coffee - 1 cup
creamer - 1 tsp
fudge - 2 pieces (2 oz)
(PM) martini, 4 oz - 2
olives - 4
crackers, butter - 5 or 6
cheese dip - 2 or 3 tbsp
nuts, mixed - handful (½ cup)
trout, broiled - 5 oz
baked potato - 1 med
sour cream - 2 tbsp
tossed salad - small
Italian dressing - 2 tbsp
croutons - 2 tbsp
ice cream, vanilla - ¾ cup
(Snack) milk, whole - 1 cup
brownie - 1 small

Total underlined items (fat): _20_ servings
Total circled items (saturated fat): _17_ servings

fewer total circled items (saturated fat) on Day Four?

Sound nutrition knowledge and food habit awareness will assist you in working towards desired dietary change. A general understanding of your individual nutrient needs (eg, protein, carbohydrate, fat), coupled with the ability to observe your own food habits can pave the road to nutritional health and well-being.

Sources of Saturated Fat

Food	Approximate % Saturated Fat	Comments
Red Meat - Prime grade	50–60	
Choice grade	35–40	
Good grade	25–35	
Young beef	least of all grades	
Ground Meat - Regular	30–35	
Lean	20–25	
Extra lean	15–20	
Prepared Meats -		
Sausage	35–40	Some special brands (made from soy-
Precooked sausage	10–15	beans) do not contain any
Cured meat	35–40	saturated fat or cholesterol.
Luncheon meat	35–40	
Poultry Chicken	30–35	Remove skin (rich in fat).
Turkey	30–35	
Fish	low	
Cheese - Hard	45–50	Alternatives now available with low/no
Part skim	30	saturated fat and/or cholesterol con-
Processed food, spread	20–30	tents include: skim-milk cheeses, Count Down, Cheezola, Chef's Delight,
Cream	50–60	Dorman's Tilsit, and others.
Milk - Whole	3.5	
Low-fat	2	
Skim	0	
Ice Cream	10–20	
Ice Milk	10	
Cream	50–60	
Butter	55	
Palm Oil		Many food labels indicate only
Coconut Oil	high	"vegetable oil," which includes
Cocoa Butter		highly saturated products.
Shortening	high	These are common ingredients in
Hydrogenated Oils		processed foods—since they are more stable than unsaturated fats.
Nuts	varying	Dry roasted and raw nuts do not con- tain cholesterol, and have less total fat than those roasted in oil.
Fried Foods	varying	Unless otherwise labeled, most com- mercially fried foods are prepared in hydrogenated oils.

DAY FIVE

VITAMIN VERIFICATION

STEP 1: THE SECURITY BLANKET MYTH

On the chart below, list any vitamin supplement(s) you may take. Include brand name(s) and milligrams/grams per supplement. Indicate by check (✔) whether you take the supplement(s) on a regular or sporadic basis and if it is medically or self-prescribed. Record price per purchase in the cost column (eg, $5.95 per 100 pills). Finally, in the comments column, explain why you are taking each supplement (eg, to combat fatigue, prevent common colds, etc).

Vitamin and Dosage	Brand Name	Taken Daily (✔)	Taken Other (✔)	Prescribed Self (✔)	Prescribed Medically (✔)	Cost	Comments

Americans spend over a billion dollars each year on self-prescribed vitamin supplements. Yet, for the majority of individuals, supplementation is unnecessary. Because of common vitamin misconceptions, many Americans continuously succumb to vitamin sales pitches and "health with vitamins" promotions. Let's take a look at some of the popular myths about vitamins, and then examine the facts.

Myth: Vitamin supplements serve as an insurance policy for guaranteed health, even for those consuming an unbalanced diet.

Fact: There are approximately 55 nutrients necessary for proper body function and optimal nutritional status, including a variety of vitamins. Minute quantities of the known vitamins are required in the regulation of body processes. The normal healthy individual who eats a wide variety of nutritious foods can easily obtain all of the necessary vitamins. Vitamin supplementation cannot make up for an inadequate intake of other nutrients. After all, vitamin supplements do not provide the protein, carbohydrate, fat, or minerals we need for growth and health. Nor does a vitamin supplement supply fiber. Also, our foods may provide certain essential minerals that science has not yet identified. Thus, the surest, simplest guide to adequate nutrient intake is the selection of a variety of foods from the basic food groups. Because vitamins occur in differing amounts in the vast array of foods now available, variety in food selection is essential.

STEP 2: THE DEFICIENT FOOD SUPPLY MYTH

Myth: Foods available in our supermarkets cannot provide us with adequate amounts of the necessary nutrients.

Fact: We now know more than ever before about the nutrient content of our food supply and about our individual nutrient needs. The problem is not that our foods are nutrient deficient. Rather, our food choices are inappropriate, the inclusion of vitamin-rich foods is insufficient, and methods of home preparation are vitamin destructive. Commercially available foods can easily meet all of the nutrient needs of the wise shopper and cook. You may want to use the chart on page 27 as a helpful guide toward more selective shopping and in the proper preparation of vitamin-rich foods; post it on your kitchen cabinet or wallboard for easy referral during menu planning and food preparation.

Fresh fruits and vegetables are at their nutritional peak immediately after harvesting. They should be rapidly transported from the garden, and handled and stored properly in order to preserve both the quality of freshness and the quantity of nutrients. To best preserve the nutrients in fresh produce, try these tips:

- Buy only the freshest produce; nutrients are lost when fruits and vegetables are old, wilted, or bruised.
- Buy only in-season produce, and only as much as will be eaten.
- Darker colored vegetables are usually richer in nutrients (eg, dark green lettuce leaves contain more vitamins than paler leaves).
- Ripen tomatoes at room temperature and use immediately to avoid large losses of vitamin C.
- Leave vegetables in their husks, pods, or skins until immediately prior to cooking or consumption.
- Keep vegetables in plastic wrap in the crisper section of the refrigerator to prevent wilting.

STEP 3: THE DEPLETED SOIL MYTH

Complete the following questionnaire about your own produce purchasing habits by checking (✓) the appropriate boxes.

	Yes	No
1) I usually buy organic fruits.	☐	☐
2) I usually buy organic vegetables.	☐	☐
3) I purchase my organic produce from health food stores or farmer's markets.	☐	☐

	More	Less
4) I usually pay _____ for my organic produce than I would pay for produce from local supermarkets.	☐	☐

The fact that many Americans spend a good share of their food dollars on so-called organic fruits and vegetables is due to the popular misconception that organically fertilized soil is nutritionally superior to today's nutrient-poor soil. Actually, organic fertilizer has been shown to contain dangerous amounts of natural toxins, and organic produce often sells at five times the cost of safer nonorganic produce. More information on organic foods is given on Day Twenty-Seven.

Vitamin	Best Food Sources	Additional Tips
A	Fish-liver oils, liver, margarine, butter, whole and fortified milk, cheese, cream, egg yolk, dark green leafy vegetables, bright yellow fruits and vegetables.	Cooking vegetables increases the availability; deeper color in vegetables indicates richer amounts.
D	Fish-liver oils, fortified milk.	Exposure of skin to sunlight creates this vitamin; milk should be labeled as "fortified with vitamin D."
E	Vegetable oils, margarine, nuts, dried beans and peas, wheat germ.	Destroyed by light, air, and in bleaching of flour; avoid excessive intake of vegetable oils.
K	Dark green leafy vegetables, cauliflower, cereals.	Destroyed by light, acids and antibiotic drug therapy.
C	Citrus fruits, tomatoes, strawberries, cantaloupe, cabbage, broccoli, potatoes, green peppers.	Destroyed by contact with copper, iron, heat, air; dissolves easily in cooking water and if food source is finely chopped.
B_1 (Thiamin)	Lean pork, organ meats, whole grains, wheat germ, dried beans and peas, milk, peanuts.	Destroyed by heat and air; dissolves easily in cooking water.
B_2 (Riboflavin)	Milk, organ meats, lean meats, eggs, dark green leafy vegetables.	Destroyed by ultraviolet light (sunlight); store in cool, dark place.
Niacin	Lean meat, poultry, fish, organ meats, whole grains, dark green leafy vegetables, peanuts, milk.	May be lost with excessive heat, air, light exposure.
B_6 (Pyridoxine)	Wheat germ, lean meat, organ meats, milk, whole grains, legumes, corn.	Destroyed by heat; use of oral contraceptives increases requirement.
Folic Acid	Organ meats, dark green leafy vegetables, legumes.	Destroyed by heat during long storage; lost in acid medium, as when cooked in vinegar.
B_{12}	All foods of animal origin (meat, milk, dairy products), specially prepared fermented yeasts and soy products.	Destroyed by air and light; strict vegetarians must include the special yeasts and/or soy products.

Note that the nutritive value of all produce is influenced by the following factors: genetic makeup of the plant, soil, climate, harvesting, season, storage methods, and handling techniques.

Myth: Our soil is nutritionally deficient, making the foods grown in it low in vitamin content.

Fact: Only very slight variations in the nutritive value of crops are due to soil quality. The nutritive value of plants is influenced more by genetic makeup than by the fertility of the soil. The protein, carbohydrate, fat, vitamin, and fiber content of a plant is controlled by the plant's particular genetic composition, rather than by the soil. On the other hand, a high mineral content in the soil may be reflected in the crops, but this is usually of little significance. However, soil rich in certain minerals can produce plants with undesirably high contents of some specific minerals; the consumption of excessive amounts of certain minerals can cause toxic side effects. (Day Six discusses minerals in more detail.)

STEP 4: THE ENERGY BOOSTER MYTH

Myth: Vitamins supply extra energy, vim and vigor to cure "that run-down feeling."

Fact: Energy is supplied by food in the form of calories. Protein, carbohydrate, and fat provide calories, while vitamins, minerals, and water are all calorie-free. Since vitamins do not provide calories, they do not furnish the body with energy. Some vitamins aid in the conversion of foods to usable energy, but "that run-down feeling" usually is not caused by a vitamin deficiency. To be energetic and full of vigor usually requires more than a vitamin supplement can provide.

During Day Five, take special notice of any vitamin supplements you see advertised in newspapers, magazines, store displays, or anywhere else. In the chart on page 28, record the various brand names and any proposed health benefits. Indicate the cost per purchase as well.

Brand Name	Where Advertised	Proposed Benefits	Cost

STEP 5: THE NATURAL IS BETTER MYTH

Indicate whether you think the following statements are True or False:

____ 1) Natural vitamins are nutritionally superior to those synthesized in the laboratory.

____ 2) Natural vitamin supplements are free of synthetic ingredients.

____ 3) Natural vitamin supplements can cost five times as much as their synthetic counterparts.

Myth: Vitamin preparations labeled as "natural" are better than the synthetic products.

Fact: The fact that many people purchase the expensive vitamin supplements marked "natural" instead of the cheaper synthetic preparations is due to the common misconception that natural vitamins are both superior to and free of synthetics. Actually, natural and synthetic vitamins have the same chemical structure, whether synthesized in the laboratory, extracted from an animal or plant food, or consumed as part of an animal or plant food. Quite surprisingly, synthetic ingredients are often present in the so-called natural supplements, since many vitamin manufacturing companies use excipients and binders such as ethylcellulose and polysorbate 80 (we will discuss additives further on Day Twenty-Eight). The body cannot distinguish between natural and synthetic structures, but your wallet can: considering the price of daily vitamin supplements—natural costing five or more times the price of most synthetics—a balanced diet seems to be the wisest method for vitamin intake. An important point to consider as well is that the effectiveness of a vitamin is controlled not by origin (natural vs synthetic), but by whether or not the body actually needs it.

STEP 6: THE MEGADOSE MYTH

A megavitamin is a vitamin preparation which provides ten or more times the recommended dietary allowance. In most cases, this is the lowest level at which symptoms of toxicity may begin to appear. However, in infants and in certain susceptible individuals, a substantially lower dosage can lead to vitamin toxicity. When vitamins are taken in large dosages, their use becomes pharmaceutical and the vitamins are then considered drugs.

Myth: Since a certain amount of vitamins will provide health benefits, huge dosages will offer an added boon to health and well-being.

Fact: The accepted guide for vitamin intake is based on the actual amounts used in the body. Extra doses of vitamins are useful only in documented deficiencies. Unneeded vitamins are either excreted, which puts a strain on the kidneys, or stored—even up to toxic levels. A disproportionate amount of any one nutrient tends to alter the function of other nutrients, and an unhealthy imbalance can occur with indiscriminate self-dosages of vitamins. Vitamin supplements may be medically prescribed for growing children, pregnant women, and individuals with specific illnesses, but for the average, healthy individual, a well-balanced diet supplies sufficient vitamins to ensure nutritional health. It is our responsibility to be able to select food wisely, in order that we may achieve the benefits of a well-balanced, vitamin-rich diet.

Use the chart below to compare some of the important functions of several vitamins with the results of an overdose of each. Remember that, for the average, healthy individual, a well-balanced diet can supply all of the vitamins necessary for health in an affordable and safe manner.

Vitamin	Energy	Major Function In: Body Cells	Body Processes	Symptoms of Overdose
A		Increases resistance to infection.	Maintains normal skin; promotes healthy eyes and eye adaptation in dim light; aids growth.	Yellow deposits on hands and feet, retarded growth, dry skin, headaches, bone pain, lack of appetite, hair loss, liver damage, death.
B_1 (Thiamin) B_2 (Riboflavin), and Niacin	Aid in energy use.		Promote healthy skin, eyes, nerves, appetite, and digestion.	Flushing and itching skin, skin disorders, liver damage, peptic ulcer, high blood sugar levels, gout.
C		Strengthens blood vessels; speeds wound healing; increases resistance to infection.	Aids in iron use.	Gastrointestinal disturbances, kidney disorders, damage to growing bones, rebound scurvy (swollen gums, loose teeth), muscle pain.
D			Promotes bone development.	Retarded physical and mental development, nausea, weakness, weight loss, kidney stones, kidney failure, high blood pressure, calcium deposits in tissue, death.
E		Antioxidant: protects cell structure in body (also retards food spoilage).		Headaches, nausea, fatigue, blurred vision, inflammation of mouth, intestinal disturbances, muscle weakness, low blood sugar levels, interference with absorption of vitamin K.
K	Involved in energy creation.		Promotes proper blood clotting.	Increased clotting (especially dangerous with certain antidote medications).
B_6 (Pyridoxine)		Involved in protein synthesis.		Interferes with certain medications.
Folic Acid		Forms red blood cells.	Prevents anemia.	Masks certain anemias; kidney damage.
B_{12}		Involved in blood formation.	Promotes growth; health of nervous system.	Liver damage.

STEP 7: THE VITAMIN C AND STRESS MYTH

Many Americans tend to avoid those foods which are rich sources of vitamin C. Yet supplementation with vitamin C, often in doses ten to 200 times the recommended dietary allowances, has become quite popular.

In the list below check (✔) those items which you think can provide the recommended dietary allowance of vitamin C for the normal, healthy adult:

_____ a medium orange
_____ 1000 mg capsule of vitamin C
_____ ½ cup raw cabbage
_____ 2 gm capsule of vitamin C
_____ fresh fruit salad: ¼ grapefruit, ¼ cantaloupe, ½ cup strawberries, ¼ cup pineapple
_____ a large baked potato
_____ ½ cup broccoli

All of the above selections could provide the adult recommended dietary allowance for vitamin C of 60 milligrams per day. This recommended dosage is enough to meet normal bodily demands, with a generous margin of safety as well.

Myth: Massive doses of vitamin C are effective in treating both physical and psychological stress, including symptoms of the common cold.

Fact: There is no evidence to suggest that vitamin C in amounts exceeding the recommended dietary allowances can be of physical benefit—in coping with stress or preventing the common cold. The popular claims depicting increased bodily needs for vitamin C during periods of physical and psychological stress are based on the insignificant results of inconclusive animal studies. And the claims for increased needs have yet to be substantiated by studies on normal, healthy humans. Stress is currently a popular health issue, one which many "health with vitamins" promoters have successfully cashed in on. The possibility of a relationship between vitamin C intake and the common cold has been the subject of public controversy for quite a few years. However, most nutritionists and physicians do not believe that large doses of vitamin C are effective in decreasing the incidence, severity, or lifespan of the common cold and related infections. The subject requires further study, and the safety of prolonged ingestion of excessive doses of vitamin C is questionable (see chart in Step 6). Vitamin

C need not be taken in excessively large amounts, but lack of sufficient vitamin C in the diet can be detrimental to overall health. The influence of vitamin C in the absorption of iron is of special importance, since iron is difficult to absorb and is commonly deficient in the American diet (more about iron on Day Six). Again, a well-balanced diet can provide the normal, healthy individual with all of the essential nutrients required for optimal health and well-being—including those nutrients important during periods of increased physical and psychological stress.

STEP 8: VITAMIN C IN YOUR DIET

Do you obtain your recommended dietary allowance of vitamin C each day? Use your Nutri-Plan diet diary along with Appendix B and a nutrient values chart (see Appendix C) in order to determine whether you met your vitamin C needs through your food intake on Day Four. In the chart on page 31, list your food and beverage intake and the amounts for Day Four. Then determine the approximate milligrams of vitamin C per serving, and total your day's intake. Compare this total to your individual recommended dietary allowance (approximately 60 milligrams per day—see Appendix B).

STEP 9: DAY FIVE PLAN

Continue to record everything you eat and drink in your Nutri-Plan diet diary. For Day Five, continue to be aware of your intake of protein, carbohydrate, and fat. Try to approximate your personal needs, and to select foods wisely. Also, make sure your diet is a vitamin-rich one. You can refer to the chart given in Step 2 during meal planning and preparation. Be especially aware of your intake of foods high in vitamin C. Remember, vitamin supplements are an unnecessary expense when your diet is well-balanced and includes a wide variety of nutritious foods.

At the end of Day Five, complete another chart totaling your vitamin C intake using the methods you utilized in Step 8. Compare this total to the total for Day Four. Can you see any improvement over Day Four (Step 8)? Did you obtain your recommended dietary allowance on Day Five?

The ability to identify vitamin-rich foodstuffs, coupled with the effort to prepare these foods properly and to consume adequate amounts every day, helps to ensure a well-balanced and health-promoting diet.

Day Four

Food and Amounts	Vitamin C (mg)

Total Vitamin C:_____ mg
Your Individual Recommended Dietary
Allowance:_____ mg

DAY SIX

MINDING MINERALS

STEP 1: TRUTH ABOUT MINERALS

Do you think that the following statement is True or False?

True False   Our bodies need so many minerals
□   □   in such differing amounts that the only way to obtain all that we need is through supplementation.

Although vitamins are the more common dietary supplement, American consumers have become increasingly concerned with the importance of proper dietary intake of minerals as well. Like vitamins, minerals occur in tiny, yet sufficient quantities in our foods. A balanced, varied diet can easily fulfill the daily needs of a normal, healthy individual for those minerals essential for health.

Minerals account for 4% to 5% of total body weight. This means that a female weighing 120–125 pounds carries approximately five pounds of minerals in her body. Yet, we need not choke down five pounds of mineral pills and powders every day in order to meet our needs.

STEP 2: MINERALS DEFINED

The 17 minerals now known to be essential to man perform two basic functions:

1) Minerals help to build the skeleton and all soft tissues.
2) Minerals regulate body systems (eg, heartbeat, blood clotting, oxygen transport, nerve conduction, etc).

However, the 17 minerals are separated into two categories not by function, but by size:

Macrominerals—Minerals needed by the body each day in amounts greater than 100 milligrams are known as macrominerals. The seven macrominerals are:

- Calcium •Sodium •Potassium •Sulfur
  •Phosphorus •Chloride •Magnesium

Microminerals—Those minerals needed by the body in daily amounts no greater than a few milligrams are called microminerals, or trace elements. The ten trace elements are:

- Iron •Copper •Zinc •Chromium
  •Selenium •Manganese •Iodine •Cobalt
  •Fluorine •Molybdenum

The body also contains minute quantities of minerals not yet known to be essential for growth and health in man. Some of these so-called nonessential minerals include:

- Aluminum •Tin •Barium •Mercury
  •Silver •Lead •Gold

Some of these nonessential minerals can prove to be poisonous in certain amounts. Two common examples to illustrate the possibility of toxicity are:

Mercury—Swordfish and tuna were found to contain undesirably high levels of mercury, and commercial sales were banned; studies later indicated that a protective mineral, selenium, is also present in these fish, and their safety is now accepted.

Lead—Poisoning from this mineral has proven fatal for many children, usually due to the ingestion of chips of leaded paint; the use of lead-based paint is now banned in this country.

Considering the importance of minerals for proper body functioning, how much do you think that four to five pounds of these essential elements would cost, if purchased in a typical store? 10¢? $10? $100? More? Actually, purchase of your body's mineral needs would probably only cost you about ten cents! (This does not, however, include the price of any silver or gold you may have in your teeth!)

STEP 3: MINERAL DEFICIENCIES

Do you include the following items in your diet every day? You may want to refer to your Nutri-Plan diet diary, Days One through Five, to confirm your answers.

☐ Iodized salt
☐ Meat, legumes, dried fruit, or dark green leafy vegetables
☐ Milk, cheese, or yogurt

Although your body's mineral needs can be met through a well-balanced diet containing a variety of mineral-rich foodstuffs, in special circumstances certain mineral supplements are required. The three minerals which are often obtained in inadequate amounts are:

•Iodine •Iron •Calcium

Iodine—In certain geographic locations, iodine is found in insufficient quantities in the soil and water supply. A diet deficient in this mineral results in a goiter, an overworked thyroid gland, sometimes enlarged up to 15 times the normal size. Goiter is one of the most common deficiency diseases present in the world today. It is relatively rare in this country, however, due to the fact that our government mandated the addition of iodine to table salt—and we tend to consume more than enough salt (as you will see on Day Fifteen).

Iron—A deficiency in this mineral is a common world problem, and is quite prevalent in American women and children. The high incidence of iron deficiency is due to several factors, including the following:

• Iron is difficult to absorb from food.
• Iron is present only in very small quantities in our foods.
• Most iron-rich foods are unpopular items (eg, liver, dried beans, figs, spinach).
• Women and children need extra iron, due to the increased demands from menstrual blood loss and tissue growth; pregnancy also increases iron needs, largely due to fetal demands.

Ordinary diets are often unable to supply enough iron to meet these increased demands. Therefore, a confirmed deficiency usually requires iron supplementation. Iron supplements should be taken only if prescribed by a physician.

Calcium—American adults are often negligent in meeting dietary calcium requirements. Although the need for calcium does not decrease during adulthood, many people eliminate milk consumption soon after the teen years. Osteoporosis is a disease in which calcium is lost from the bones, leading to easy fracture and joint disorders. Believed to be caused in part by inadequate calcium intake, osteoporosis is quite common in elderly Americans, especially women.

STEP 4: MINERAL TOXICITY

It is not only possible to ingest an overdose of the nonessential minerals (such as mercury or lead), but in large amounts, the essential minerals can also prove to be quite toxic. Would you want to endanger your health by taking unnecessarily large dosages of the minerals below? Consider these dangerous symptoms of mineral overdoses:

Calcium—kidney stones, deposits in soft tissues
Potassium—muscle weakness, irregular heartbeat
Iron—deposits in liver, lungs, heart
Manganese—tremor, loss of coordination
Copper—deposits in liver, brain, kidney, eyes
Zinc—iron losses from liver
Selenium—gastrointestinal disorders, lung irritation
Molybdenum—diarrhea, anemia, depressed growth, gout-like syndrome

Mineral supplements are often expensive and, unless prescribed for a diagnosed deficiency, are usually unnecessary. Excessive doses of minerals, like megadoses of vitamins, are useless and can prove to be dangerous. An overemphasis on vitamins and minerals forms a strong base for food faddism.

Remember that foods supply us with a combination of nutrients (protein, carbohydrate, fat, vitamins, minerals, and water), but mineral supplements do not. And our food supply may even provide essential minerals which are still undiscovered. Avoid self-prescribed mineral supplements. They can be as detrimental to your health as they are to your budget.

STEP 5: MINERAL DUTIES

As stated earlier, the 17 essential minerals perform two basic functions:

1) Minerals help to build the skeleton and all soft tissues.
2) Minerals regulate body systems (eg, heartbeat, blood clotting, oxygen transport, nerve conduction, etc).

The specific functions of the nonessential minerals are under investigation, but so far none have been shown to be essential for human health.

A look at the chart below may help you to understand some of the specific functions of the essential nutrients. Pay close attention to the side notes as well.

Mineral	Function(s)
Calcium	99% present in bones and teeth to provide structure Other 1% vital to nerves, muscles, blood
Phosphorus	Present with calcium in bones and teeth Important for body energy Note: Regular use of antacids can lead to phosphorus depletion.
Sodium	Helps to maintain body fluid balance Note: Possible correlation between excessive sodium consumption and high blood pressure is under investigation; the average American diet supplies over 5 times the needed amount.
Chloride	Present in gastric juice Important in digestion
Potassium	Helps to maintain body fluid balance Important for healthy nerves and muscles Note: Deficiency may occur with use of certain diuretic ("water pill") medications.
Magnesium	Essential to nerves and muscles Note: Deficiency may occur during postsurgical and chronic illness, or with alcoholism.
Sulfur	Important for protein utilization Essential component in certain vitamins
Iron	Important in oxygen transport Note: Significant losses occur with menstrual blood loss and during blood formation, the greatest demands for iron occurring in pregnant women, women of childbearing ages, infants, and children; deficiency can result in anemia.
Manganese	Necessary for tendon and bone structure Note: Deficiency unknown in man.
Copper	Important in red blood cell formation, especially during infancy
Iodine	Essential to thyroid gland Deficiency results in goiter (enlarged thyroid gland) Note: Use of iodized salt can prevent a deficiency state.
Zinc	Important in transport of carbon dioxide Important for growth Deficiency results in loss of taste sensation and poor wound healing Note: Deficiency can occur in strict vegetarians.
Cobalt	Essential component of vitamin B_{12} Note: Deficiency can occur in strict vegetarians.
Chromium	Important in blood sugar regulation Deficiency results in diabetes-like condition
Fluorine	Contributes to formation of strong teeth Can reduce incidence of tooth decay, especially in children Note: Possible role in the prevention of osteoporosis (bone disease common in the elderly) currently under investigation.
Selenium	Works with vitamin E Note: Excessive intake can cause serious health disorders.
Molybdenum	Important in protein metabolism Note: Deficiency unknown in man, but excesses can cause a gout-like syndrome and copper deficiency.

STEP 6: FOOD SOURCES OF MINERALS

Use the information below to help guide you in the selection of mineral-rich foodstuffs. You may want to post this handy chart on a kitchen cabinet or wallboard for easy referral during menu planning.

Mineral	Best Food Sources
Calcium	Milk and milk products Sardines Green leafy vegetables (except spinach and chard*)
Phosphorus	Meat, poultry, fish Eggs Whole grains
Sodium	Table salt Most processed foods Meats, poultry, fish, milk, eggs
Chloride	Table salt Most processed foods
Potassium	Bananas, citrus fruits, melon, strawberries Tomatoes, potatoes Lean meats Bran, oatmeal
Magnesium	Dried beans and peas Nuts Green leafy vegetables Whole grains
Sulfur	Eggs Meat Milk, cheese Nuts, dried beans and peas
Iron†	Liver Meats, dried beans and peas Clams, oysters Dried fruits
Manganese	Bran Coffee, Tea Nuts, dried beans and peas
Copper	Organ meats Shellfish Nuts, dried beans and peas
Iodine	Iodized table salt Seafood
Zinc	Meat, poultry, fish Egg yolk Milk
Cobalt	Meat Eggs Dairy products
Chromium	Liver Whole grains
Fluorine	Fish Tea Fluoridated water
Selenium	Foods grown in selenium-rich soils Seafood Whole grains
Molybdenum	Meat Whole grains Dried beans and peas

*Certain components in the plants bind calcium so that the body is unable to absorb it properly.
†Only these few foods contain a useful and well-absorbed amount of iron.

STEP 7: CALCIUM IN YOUR DIET

Do you obtain your recommended dietary allowance of calcium each day? Use your Nutri-Plan diet diary along with Appendix B and a nutrient values chart (see Appendix C) in order to determine whether you met your calcium needs through your food intake on Day Five. In the chart on page 37, list your food and beverage intake and the amounts for Day Five. Then determine the approximate milligrams of calcium per serving, and total your day's intake. Compare this total to your individual recommended dietary allowance (approximately 800 milligrams per day—see Appendix B).

STEP 8: IRON IN YOUR DIET

Do you obtain your recommended dietary allowance of iron each day? Use your Nutri-Plan diet diary along with Appendix B and a nutrient values chart (see Appendix C) in order to determine whether you met your iron needs through your food intake on Day Five. In the chart on page 38, list your food and beverage intake and the amounts for Day Five. Then determine the approximate milligrams of iron per serving, and total your day's intake. Compare this total to your individual recommended dietary allowance (approximately 10 to 18 milligrams per day—see Appendix B).

Note: Iron is difficult for the body to absorb from food. Iron absorption is enhanced, however, in the presence of:

- Hemoglobin—found in red meats.
- Vitamin C—best food sources include citrus fruits, tomatoes, strawberries, cantaloupe, cabbage, broccoli, potatoes, and green peppers.

Thus, to insure the optimal assimilation of dietary iron, you should include a serving of meat or a vitamin C-rich food at each meal. Use the following formula to assist you in planning meals which supply significant amounts of readily absorbable iron:

Meal Includes:	Iron Rich Food	+ Plus	Meat Serving
	_____		_____
	/ Vitamin C-Rich Food		
	Or _____		

Day Five

Food and Amounts	Calcium (mg)

Total Calcium: _____mg
Your Individual Recommended Dietary Allowance: _____mg

Day Five

Food and Amounts	Iron (mg)

Total Iron: _____ mg
Your Individual Recommended Dietary Allowance: _____ mg

STEP 9: DAY SIX PLAN

Continue to record everything you eat and drink in your Nutri-Plan diet diary. For Day Six, continue to be aware of your intake of protein, carbohydrate, and fat and try to make your diet a vitamin-rich one; you can refer to the second chart from Day Five during meal planning and preparation. Try to include mineral-rich foods in your diet, too. You can refer to the chart given in Step 6 to assist you in food selection. Pay special attention to the calcium and iron contents of your food choices. In most cases mineral supplements, like vitamin supplements, are an unnecessary expense when your diet is well balanced and includes a wide variety of nutritious foods.

At the end of Day Six, complete another chart totaling your calcium intake and one for your iron intake. Use the methods you utilized in Steps 7 and 8, and compare these totals with the totals for Day Five. Can you see any improvement over Day Five (Steps 7 and 8)? Did you obtain your recommended dietary allowance for calcium on Day Six? How about iron?

The ability to identify mineral-rich foodstuffs, coupled with the inclusion of a wide variety of foods in the diet each day, assists in the development of a well-balanced dietary pattern which contributes to good health.

DAY SEVEN

WHAT ABOUT WATER?

STEP 1: OUR NECESSARY NUTRIENTS

During the past week you have been learning how to identify the nutrients in your foods. These 55 or so nutrients, essential to our health and well-being, fit into six major categories. List these categories below:

1) Protein _____
2) _____
3) _____
4) _____
5) _____
6) _____

Perhaps because it is not thought of as a food per se, water is the nutrient category which is most often overlooked. Actually, our bodies contain more water than anything else; water accounts for about 60% of total body weight. Water is present inside all body cells (intracellular) and bathes the outside of body cells (extracellular). Water also comprises the fluid portion of the blood.

From the following list, check (✓) the essential functions which water performs for us:

_____ Acts as the body's transportation system
_____ Helps to absorb shocks to the body
_____ Lubricates joints
_____ Carries digestive juices
_____ Cools body down and maintains body heat
_____ Removes body wastes

All of the body's chemical reactions for energy production and tissue formation require water. Water evaporation is the body's best technique for ridding itself of heat. Flushing away body wastes would not be possible without water. Water performs all of the functions in the above list quite adeptly.

We could conceivably survive for months without food, but not without water. The longest water fast on record was 17 days—and ended in death! On a hot, dry day most of us would probably be unable to survive for longer than 12 hours without replenishing lost water.

Obviously, water is an extremely useful nutrient.

STEP 2: HOW MUCH WATER?

How much water do you drink during the course of a typical day? Check (✓) the answer below that best approximates your average daily water intake:

_____ none
_____ 1–2 cups
_____ 3–5 cups
_____ 6–8 cups
_____ more than 8 cups

The American Medical Association advises us to consume a minimum of between one and two quarts of liquid every day. Forcing down eight big glasses of water every day, however, is a more uncomfortable and less practical method than simply obeying the dictates of your body. Scientific research has indicated that the brain contains an automatic thirst control center which maintains our body fluids in the necessary balance:

• When the amount of water in the body is low, we feel thirsty.
• When the amount of water in the body is too high, the kidneys work to rid the body of the excess.

Conditions which can lead to the depletion of body fluids include the following:

• Illness—Fever, sweating, and other conditions

associated with poor health can lead to dehydration and an increased need for fluids.

- Diuretic drugs—Use of "water pills" can deplete the body of fluids, plus minerals such as sodium and potassium; any weight loss achieved with diuretics can usually be attributed to loss of body water rather than body fat.
- Hot weather—Sweating is the body's own means for cooling itself and can lead to heat exhaustion and heatstroke if the lost body fluids are not replenished.
- Exercise—Myths and misbelief cause many athletes to curtail fluid intake during competition; a reasonable intake of water will not cause cramps, but will help to prevent dehydration, heat exhaustion, and heatstroke.
- Special diets—A diet high in either sodium or protein can lead to dehydration, since the kidneys require extra water in order to dilute both sodium and certain proteins before excretion.
- Alcoholic beverages—For every ounce of alcohol we drink, we need approximately eight ounces of water for proper metabolism. Drinkers should be careful when the level of water in the body is low (as in hot weather or at high altitudes) because blood volume is comparably lessened. This means that each ounce of alcohol makes up a greater percentage of the blood, and is therefore more potent. Have you ever noticed how difficult it is to quench your thirst on "the morning after?"

STEP 3: WHERE IS THE WATER?

There are many sources of water other than the kitchen tap. In fact, we can obtain a large percentage of the water we need from our foods. From the chart below, we are able to see that much of the total weight for most foods is actually water weight:

Food	Approximate Percent Water
Bread	35
Cheese	35 to 50
Meat	45 to 55
Eggs	65 to 75
Fish	65 to 75
Potatoes	80
Fruit	85
Vegetables	75 to 90
Milk	90
Fruit juices	90

So, even if you do not care for the taste of plain water, it is easy enough to obtain the liquid your body requires through your diet. Remember, too, that thirst is usually the best indication of your body's need for fluids. Let your body dictate your fluid intake:

- Drink more fluids during fever and illness. Fresh fruit and vegetable juices are nutritious alternatives to colas and ginger ale.
- Do not restrict fluid intake when taking diuretic medication. A glass of grapefruit or orange juice will help to replace any accompanying potassium losses. Use of diuretic drugs for weight loss purposes is inadvisable, as results are due to temporary fluid loss only.
- During hot weather or physical activity, be sure to replenish lost body fluids. Do not be afraid to drink water while exercising; studies have shown that athletes actually perform better and have more endurance if they continuously replace fluid losses during performance.
- Increase fluid intake when eating high protein or salty foodstuffs. Cheese and crackers really do need to be washed down with a beverage! And moderation in protein and salt intake is a wise idea anyway, for a number of reasons related to overall health (see Day Two and Day Fifteen).
- Keep in mind the fact that alcoholic beverages can lead to dehydration. Athletic performance can be hindered when beer or other alcohol is the beverage chosen to quench thirst during activity. Less alcohol and more mixer can help to prevent "morning after" dry mouth, and may lessen that tipsy feeling on your next plane flight!

STEP 4: SPECIAL DRINKS— ALCOHOLIC BEVERAGES

How many alcoholic beverages (beer, wine, hard liquor, liqueurs) do you drink during a typical day? You can refer to your Nutri-Plan diet diary, Days One through Six, before checking (✔) the answer from the list below which best approximates your average daily intake of alcohol:

____ none
____ 1 drink (12 oz beer, 4 oz wine, 1½ oz hard liquor or liqueur)
____ 2 to 3 drinks
____ more than 3 drinks

Alcoholic beverages are an expensive source of fluids, but form an integral component of the social lives of most Americans. And, in moderate amounts, alcohol may actually provide certain health benefits. Remember that a moderate daily intake of alcohol is one of the seven health habits.

Research has also indicated that alcohol may play a beneficial role in the prevention of cardiovascular disease. For many people, alcohol helps to relieve tensions and alleviate stress.

The key to alcohol consumption is moderation. Two or three drinks per day is considered by most to be a moderate amount, but for many individuals a lesser amount is more desirable. "Light" beers and dry wines can serve as sociable, yet low calorie choices.

STEP 5: SPECIAL DRINKS— CAFFEINE BEVERAGES

How many cups of coffee and/or tea do you drink during a typical day? Again, refer to your Nutri-Plan diet diary, Days One through Six, before checking (✔) the answer from the list below which best approximates your average daily intake of coffee and/or tea:

_____ none
_____ 1 cup
_____ 2 to 4 cups
_____ 5 to 6 cups
_____ 7 to 10 cups
_____ more than 10 cups

Coffee, tea, cocoa, and soft drinks such as cola and root beer are popular drinks, yet all contain caffeine, which is actually an addictive drug. Your daily intake of these products should be of some concern, since caffeine is contraindicated for:

• Children—acts as a stimulant and may enhance hyperactivity
• Pregnant women—is transferred to the fetus
• Sensitive individuals—side effects include shakiness, insomnia, nervousness, irritability, with headache and fatigue upon withdrawal.

After all, caffeine is a drug, and we should deal with it as such. The following products may also contain caffeine (when in doubt, check the label):

• Soft drinks (Mountain Dew, Dr. Pepper, etc)
• Over-the-counter headache remedies (Excedrin, Anacin, etc)
• Over-the-counter "diet pills" (Dexatrim, Dietac, Appedrine, Prolamine, etc)
• Over-the-counter "wake-up pills" (No-Doz, Quick Pep, etc)
• "Decaffeinated" drinks (usually not 100% caffeine-free)
• Herbal teas (some contain caffeine)

You may want to refer to the average amounts of caffeine given in the following chart in order to determine the approximate quantities of caffeine in your favorite beverages or medications.

Product	Caffeine (in milligrams)
Coffee, brewed	100 to 150/cup
Coffee, instant	60 to 100/cup
Coffee, decaffeinated	2 to 5/cup
Tea	45 to 75/cup
Cocoa	13/5 ounces
Milk chocolate	6/ounce
Dr. Pepper	60/12 ounces
Mr. Pibb	55/12 ounces
Mountain Dew	50/12 ounces
Tab	45/12 ounces
Coca Cola	40/12 ounces
RC Cola	35/12 ounces
Pepsi	35/12 ounces
Diet Pepsi	35/12 ounces
Pepsi Light	35/12 ounces
Caffedrine tablet	250
Vivarin tablet	200
Double-E Alertness capsule	180
Quick-Pep tablet	150
Prolamine capsule	140
No-Doz tablet	100
Excedrin	65
Vanquish	35
Empirin Compound	30
Anacin	30
Dristan	15

STEP 6: SPECIAL DRINKS— SPORTS DRINKS

Contrary to popular belief, athletes do not obtain any special benefits from consumption of so-called sports drinks. Most of the claims for these beverages are made by trainers, coaches, and of course the sports drink manufacturers. The highly sweetened varieties and sugar-rich "protein" shakes can cause stomach cramping and gastrointestinal distress.

The best beverage for the athlete, or anyone involved in physical activity, is water. Why pay exorbitant prices for unnecessary beverages when your fluid needs can be obtained so easily (and cheaply!) from the good old water fountain? This, and many other myths common among athletes, will be discussed further on Day Twenty-Five.

STEP 7: SPECIAL DRINKS—DIET DRINKS

Liquid diets for the weight conscious are costly, commonly ineffective in achieving permanent results, and some have actually proven fatal. Liquid diet beverages merely serve as a sweet, vitamin-fortified milk drink that can be substituted for a meal (or meals). Nutritionally and economically, it is wiser to eat a calorically comparable, well-balanced meal. To illustrate this fact, compare the following "diet lunch" menus. Which one would satisfy your palate—as well as meet your nutritional needs, allot for your weight loss efforts, and keep your budget in balance?

Liquid Diet Lunch (10 oz)
"Slender Wonder"—
ingredients: skim milk, sugar, sodium
   caseinate, corn oil, cocoa, artificial flavors,
   salt
calories: 225
protein: 11 grams
carbohydrate: 34 grams
fat: 5 grams
notable vitamins: riboflavin
iron: trace
calcium: 200 milligrams
cost per serving: $1.19
Others Group: sugar, sodium (salt), fat

De-Light-Full Lunch (2 slices)
"Health Pizza"—
ingredients: whole wheat crust, low-fat cheese,
   tomatoes, mushrooms, green peppers, bean
   sprouts, seasonings
calories: 110 per slice = 220 per serving
protein: 15 grams
carbohydrate: 34 grams
fat: 4 grams
notable vitamins: A, C, B (including folic acid)
iron: 1.8 milligrams
calcium: 250 milligrams
cost per serving: 65¢
Others Group: negligible

Another popular beverage amongst weight-watchers, and currently a topic of much controversy, is the diet soft drink. In the 1960s, these beverages contained the non-nutritive sweetener cyclamate, use of which was banned in this country when laboratory tests indicated a possible carcinogenic (cancer-causing) role. Saccharin is currently the non-nutritive sweetener added to diet soft drinks, but it too has been accused of inducing cancerous tumors. Research on both of these sweeteners has not provided conclusive evidence of any potential dangers to humans consuming moderate amounts. The use of cyclamate is allowed in Canada and most European nations, and saccharin is still allowed in this country due to the amount of protest the proposed ban aroused. Products which contain saccharin must carry the following statement:

"Use of this product may be hazardous to your health. This product contains saccharin which has been determined to cause cancer in laboratory animals."

Research continues, and a moderate intake of diet soft drinks may prove harmless. However, remember that these beverages are nutritionally barren, ridiculously overpriced, and often contain a considerable amount of caffeine.

*   *   *

All in all, the wisest beverage choices are those which provide essential nutrients, yet damage neither health nor budget. Mineral water is a popular alternative to tap water, but the high cost is not accompanied by any special health benefits; the mineral content depends entirely on the source, just like the mineral content of your tap water. Soda water is usually less expensive, and can be sipped on as is or mixed with various other beverages. Milk, fruit juices, and vegetable juices provide a variety of nutrients, and can be included in the diet in many different forms. Yogurt shakes, fruit whips, and vegetable coolers can all serve to quench your thirst without ruining your waistline, health, or food budget! Recipes for low-calorie, nutrient-rich drinks are included in Days Twenty-One and Twenty-Three.

STEP 8: WATER IN YOUR DIET

Do you include enough fluid in your diet each day to provide for optimal health? Use your Nutri-Plan diet diary to determine the number of cups of fluid you drank on Day Six. In the chart on page 45, list your beverage intake and the amounts in ounces for Day Six. Then total your day's intake. If you drank any water (which you probably did not include on your Nutri-Plan diet diary), estimate the amount and add it to the total. Divide the total by 16 (to determine the number of cups of fluid). Considering the water contained in your food intake as well, do you think you consumed enough fluid (6 to 8 cups) on Day Six? Next, circle any beverage listed in your chart which fits into one of the following categories:

• Alcoholic Beverage
• Caffeine Beverage
• "Sports" Drink
• Diet Drink

Total the amount (in ounces) consumed for these less nutritious beverage choices, and again divide the total by 16; how many cups did you consume?

Day Six

Beverages	Amount in Ounces

Total Amount: _____ ounces

+ Any (estimated) Water Intake: _____ ounces   ÷ 16 = _____ cups

Total Amount Circled Beverages: _____ ounces ÷ 16 = _____ cups

STEP 9: DAY SEVEN PLAN

Continue to record everything you eat and drink in your Nutri-Plan diet diary. For Day Seven, continue to be aware of your intake of protein, carbohydrate, fat, vitamins and minerals.

At the end of Day Seven, complete another chart totaling your fluid intake using the methods you utilized in Step 8. Compare these totals with the totals for Day Six. Did you include six to eight cups of liquid on Day Seven? How many cups of the less nutritious beverages did you drink on Day Seven? Would you be able to decrease this last amount, and substitute more nutritious beverages instead?

After all, water *is* an essential nutrient, and fluids in the diet are an integral aspect of nutritional health. The wise selection of a variety of nutritious beverages each day is another step toward the development of a well-balanced dietary pattern, one which brings you closer to optimal health.

DAY EIGHT

NUTRITION KNOW-HOW

STEP 1: FOOD LIKES

With the vast amount and variety of foods now available to us, it would seem next to impossible for the typical American to *not* meet his or her nutritional needs. The typical American diet supplied by the local supermarket includes all of the nutrients that the body requires—and plenty of them! Yet, not every American is "typical."

Individuality is an important aspect of nutritional needs. Do your personal tastes—your food likes and dislikes—allow for proper nutrition? List ten of your most favorite foods on the chart below, and indicate approximately how often you eat each item (eg, daily, weekly, three times per week, once a year, etc). A few samples are illustrated for you.

STEP 2: FOOD DISLIKES

Now list ten of your least favorite foods on the chart on page 48. Indicate by checking (✓) whether each item is something that you:

- Never include in your diet—(R)—and refuse to eat.
- Dislike intensely—(D)—and rarely eat, if ever.
- Simply avoid—(A)—for various reasons.

A few samples are illustrated below. Note that there may not be ten foods which you dislike. In fact, some people like everything edible!

Sample Chart

Food likes	Frequency of Consumption
1) Fresh lobster tails	once a month—during the summer only
2) Homemade pecan pie	maybe 2 × a year
3) Martini, extra dry	3 at lunch during workweek
4) Anything chocolate	1 to 2 × a month—on "binges"

Your Chart

Food Likes	Frequency of Consumption
1)	
2)	
3)	
4)	
5)	
6)	
7)	
8)	
9)	
10)	

Sample Chart

Food Dislikes	Degree of Dislike (✔)		
	(R)	(D)	(A)
1) Lima beans	✔		
2) Milk			✔
3) Alcoholic beverages, any kind			✔
4) Fish, except fried		✔	

Your Chart

Food Dislikes	Degree of Dislike (✔)		
	(R)	(D)	(A)
1)			
2)			
3)			
4)			
5)			
6)			
7)			
8)			
9)			
10)			

Compare your food dislikes with your food likes (Step 1). Do you have a taste for rich foods, or do you prefer plainer foods? Are your likes varied, or are they all similar kinds of foods? Do you tend to dislike fruits and vegetables, and refuse to eat desserts?

Every individual has different tastes for life, including tastes for food. Your personal food likes and dislikes need to be incorporated into your individual dietary pattern. After all, if you like martinis and dislike lima beans, it would be intolerable, unpleasurable, and probably impossible for you to adhere to a diet based on the latter and excluding the former!

Thus, in balancing out your diet, it is important for you to keep in mind your individual tastes. However, in selecting foods from the wide variety now available, it is also important for you to try new foods. Keep an open mind: tastes tend to change with age, and advance with the times. Remember, you might have disliked shrimp as a child, and liked peanut butter spread on pizza during your teen years!

STEP 3: STYLES AND BELIEFS

In addition to particular food likes and dislikes, your dietary patterns are also influenced by your individual lifestyles and beliefs. For some people, the way they live detracts from food intake and nutritional status (eg, the busy executive who skips lunch and indulges in several martinis every evening, the weight conscious teen who skips breakfast but nibbles on candy later on). Some people have lifestyles which regularly result in overindulgences and often lead to overweight (eg, the housewife who constantly samples her own cooking, the socialite who spends every weekend at dinner dates, brunches, and cocktail parties).

People who live alone often exist almost exclusively on convenience foods, while the pace of today's society has led others to regularly rely on fast food restaurants. Others may derive their diet from whole, natural foods grown organically or at home. Vegetarian, Kosher, macrobiotic and other cultural practices also set limitations on the nutritional intakes of many Americans.

How does your lifestyle influence your diet? Do you have any special beliefs or practices which affect your food intake? Complete the following questionnaire in order to determine the personal styles and beliefs which help to form your own dietary patterns. You may want to refer to your Nutri-Plan diet diary to assist you in answering the questions as accurately as possible. Elaborate as much as desired, and be honest with yourself!

Questionnaire

1) How does your job influence your dietary patterns?
   - How many meals and snacks do you eat at work each day? _____
   - Do you eat these meals/snacks at the office, in a restaurant, in a cafeteria, or do you go home? _____
   - Do you eat breakfast before going to work, at work, or not at all on work days? _____
   - How many coffee breaks do you take each day? _____ What do you usually eat and/or drink at this time? _____
   - Do you keep food at your desk? _____ Do you snack while working? _____
   - Do you ever utilize the food vending machines at your office? _____
     What vending machine items do you buy? _____

2) How does your home life influence your dietary patterns?
   - How many meals and snacks do you eat at home each day? _____
   - Do you eat at regular times each day? _____
   - Do you prepare your own meals? _____ Your family's meals? _____
   - Do you find yourself eating during meal preparation/clean-up? _____
   - Do you eat alone? _____ Do you eat any meals/snacks with others? _____
   - For approximately how many minutes do your meals last?
     Breakfast _____ Lunch _____ Dinner _____ Others _____
   - Approximately how many hours of television do you watch each day? _____ And, do you usually eat while watching television? _____

3) Do you have any religious and/or cultural beliefs which influence your dietary patterns?
   - Do you follow any of the following dietary practices:
     _____ Kosher
     _____ Vegetarian
     _____ Seventh Day Adventist
     _____ Macrobiotic
     _____ Other: _____
   - Due to your cultural background, do you follow a diet based on any of the following types of foods:
     _____ Chinese/Polynesian/Japanese
     _____ Italian
     _____ Spanish/Cuban
     _____ Mexican
     _____ Indian
     _____ "Soul"
     _____ Other: _____

4) Are there other lifestyle patterns and personal beliefs which influence your dietary habits:
   - Do you eat convenience foods? _____ List any which you eat regularly:
     _____
   - Do you eat so-called health foods? _____ List any which you eat regularly: _____
   - Do you eat so-called dietetic foods? _____ List any which you eat regularly: _____
   - Do you eat at fast food restaurants? _____ How often? _____
   - Do you eat at other types of restaurants? _____ List any kinds which you attend regularly (eg, seafood, steakhouse, salad bar, pancake house, ethnic, etc) and indicate approximately how often you visit each: _____

STEP 4: HEALTH AND ILLNESS

Many Americans adopt special diets for the management of specific health problems, such as:
• Overweight
• Underweight
• Diabetes
• High blood pressure
• Cardiovascular disease
• Allergies
• Ulcers
• Chronic digestive disorders
• Gout
• General recovery from illness or surgery

Health problems, especially those which incur dietary change, can distort nutritional balance. On the chart below, list the personal health problems that you may have, if any, which influence your dietary patterns, and explain briefly the dietary changes you have made. A few samples are illustrated for you.

Note the number of health problems which directly affect your diet. You may want to visit a nutritionist who can assist you in balancing your diet in spite of any necessary restrictions or alterations. Contact the Dietetics Department of your local hospital for information on how you can arrange for a nutrition counseling appointment.

STEP 5: NUTRITION KNOWLEDGE

Perhaps even more than your individual characteristics such as food likes/dislikes, lifestyles and

Sample Chart

Specific Health Problem	Dietary Adaptations
1) Diabetes	I am on an 1800 ADA diet, avoid sugar, and watch my fat intake.
2) Allergic to milk	I avoid most milk products, but am able to eat cheese.
3) Overweight	I am constantly trying to lose weight using a variety of diets.

Your Chart

Specific Health Problem	Dietary Adaptations

beliefs, or health problems, your knowledge on the subject of nutrition has a profound influence on your diet, and ultimately on your nutritional status. How much nutrition education have you been able to obtain? On the following chart, check (✔) the amount of nutrition education which you have received:

_____ I have had little or no nutrition education.

_____ I had some nutrition education in high school (eg, in home economics, science, health, or physical education class).

_____ I have attended workshops/continuing education classes on nutrition.

_____ I have taken college level course(s) in nutrition.

_____ I have a college degree in nutrition.

_____ I have done graduate work in nutrition.

Next, indicate your current interest level in the area of nutrition by checking (✔) the most appropriate frequency for each of the following statements:

Daily	Weekly	Monthly	Rarely	Never	
☐	☐	☐	☐	☐	1) I read magazine and/or newspaper articles about nutrition.
☐	☐	☐	☐	☐	2) I read books about nutrition.
☐	☐	☐	☐	☐	3) I have recently taken and/or am currently taking course(s) in nutrition.
☐	☐	☐	☐	☐	4) I discuss nutrition with others.
☐	☐	☐	☐	☐	5) I think about my own diet, the changes I can make, and the effect of diet on my health and well-being.

STEP 6: WORKING TOWARD NUTRITION KNOW-HOW

The amount of knowledge you obtain in the area of nutrition greatly influences your food choices and dietary patterns. Last week you began to learn some of the basics about nutrition and the well-balanced diet. You also began to record your food intake and eating habits in order to better visualize your own dietary patterns. And today, you began to look at some of the many different influences on your food intake.

The next step is to combine your nutrition knowledge with an understanding of your own food habits and specific dietary influences:

By combining these three factors, you are able to take an important step toward balancing your diet. You need not make any drastic changes:

- You do not have to bring a nutrition text to every meal.
- You do not have to overthrow all your old dietary habits to start anew.
- You do not have to stop eating the foods you like, nor start eating foods that you do not enjoy.
- You do not have to adopt a new religion, a different culture, or another body (one in "perfect" health).
- You do not have to get a doctoral degree (nor any sort of degree) in nutrition.

You do need to begin to incorporate some of the new knowledge you are gaining about nutrition and your own diet into an individualized and evolving dietary pattern. Thus, you should combine the following factors:

Nutrition Basics + Your Personal Eating Habits + Your Individual Dietary Influences

Eventually this combination will evolve into an individualized, health-promoting, personally enjoyable dietary plan which is part of your own particular lifestyle. All it takes is the proper attitude, plus a sufficient amount of nutrition know-how.

STEP 7: REMEMBER THE BASICS?

On Day One, you took a close look at your own diet and compared it to a chart depicting the recommended servings from the basic food groups. During Days Eleven through Fifteen, the groups will be discussed in more detail. Specific factors to consider when selecting foods from each group will

Knowledge of some basics about:		Understanding your own food habits such as:		Understanding specific dietary influences such as:
Protein		Length of mealtimes		Food likes and dislikes
Carbohydrate	+	Types of foods eaten	+	Lifestyle and beliefs
Fat		Types of hunger		Diet-related health problems
Vitamins		Feelings about food intake and		Amount of nutrition education
Minerals		hunger		
Water				

be explained, and the serving sizes for different foodstuffs will be illustrated. Thus, by choosing the appropriate number of servings each day from the basic food groups, and by including a variety of foods in your daily diet, it will soon be as easy as it is sensible for you to enjoy a well-balanced diet.

For a quick review of the basic food groups, complete the chart below. Indicate the number of daily servings you need from each group, and list some possible food sources. The Milk and Cheese Group has been completed for you. To check your answers, examine the chart given in Day One.

STEP 8: YOUR BASIC DIET

Do you think that your diet now approximates the recommended servings from each of the basic food groups? Do you think you have at least improved since Day One? Use your Nutri-Plan diet diary and the chart given in Day One to determine whether your diet included the proper number of recommended servings from each of the basic food

groups on Day Seven. In the chart on page 53, list all foods and beverages consumed on Day Seven and the amounts. Determine the approximate number of servings for each group and compare this amount to the No. Recommended Servings. Look carefully at the sample chart given below which has been completed for you; note the explanations for totaling servings eaten.

Did your diet on Day Seven include enough fruit? Vegetables? Grains? Milk and cheese? Meat and alternates? How many servings from the Others Group did you include?

STEP 9: DAY EIGHT PLAN

Continue to record everything you eat and drink in your Nutri-Plan diet diary. For Day Eight, continue to be aware of your intake of protein, carbohydrate, fat, vitamins, and minerals. Be sure that you are including enough water in your diet, either as part of your food and beverage consumption or straight from the tap.

Basic Food Group	No. Servings per Day	Food Sources
Fruit and Vegetable		
Grain		
Milk and Cheese	2 (adult), 3 (child), 4 (teen)	Milk—whole, skim, buttermilk, cheese, yogurt
Meat and Alternates		
Others		

Sample Chart

Basic Food Group	No. Recommended Servings	Foods Eaten and Amounts	No. Servings Eaten
Fruit and Vegetable	4	orange juice—½ cup apple—1 med broccoli—1 cup	4 (broccoli = ½ cup + ½ cup or 2 servings)
Grain	4	hot cereal—¾ cup wheat bread—2 sl English muffin—½	4 (½ muffin = 1 serving)
Milk and Cheese	2 (adult) 3 (child) 4 (teen)	whole milk—¼ cup (in coffee)	¼
Meat and Alternates	2	chicken, broiled—6 oz	3 (2 oz = 1 serving)
Others	—	Coffee—2 cups Sugar—2 tsp (in coffee) Donut—1 chocolate Mayonnaise—1 tsp Margarine—2 tsp Wine—3½ oz Pie, apple—1 av slice Ice cream, vanilla—½ cup	11 (simply count each serving of food or beverage as one serving and ignore serving sizes)

At the end of Day Eight, complete another chart totaling your basic food group servings using the methods you utilized in Step 8. Were there any groups for which you did not obtain the recommended number of daily servings? How many servings from the Others Group did you include on Day Eight? Did you have fewer servings of the Others Group foods on Day Eight than on Day Seven?

To ensure that your diet is balanced, simply select a variety of foods from the basic food groups and include them in your daily diet in the recommended amounts. In no time at all, wise food selection will become a habit—one you can live with, healthfully!

Day Seven

Basic Food Group	No. Recommended Servings	Foods Eaten and Amounts	No. Servings Eaten
Fruit and Vegetable	4		
Grain	4		
Milk and Cheese	2 (adult) 3 (child) 4 (teen)		
Meat and Alternates	2		
Others	—		

DAY NINE

COUNTING CALORIES

STEP 1: HOW FAT ARE WE?

Americans read thousands of books every year in desperate search of a cure for excess poundage. We think about and discuss the topic of weight loss incessantly, yet the results are not often in our favor: more than one third of our population is overweight. The majority of those who are seriously overweight (obese) are middle-aged, usually because it takes time for the excess fat deposits to build, and often because of the sedentary lifestyle which most adults settle into.

From the list below, check (ν) the disorders which you think might occur more frequently in the overweight:

____ heart disease
____ high blood pressure
____ diabetes
____ arthritis
____ gallbladder disease
____ respiratory ailments
____ fertility/pregnancy problems

All of these disorders are more likely to develop in overweight persons than in those of normal weight. Overweight people also tend to have abnormal skin conditions, varicose veins, and are often considered to be surgical risks. And the greater the degree of overweight, the shorter the life expectancy. However, overweight persons can diminish the probability of developing these health problems and can increase life expectancy simply by attaining and maintaining proper body weight... and the key to weight control is calorie control.

STEP 2: SCALE WATCHING

Although most overweight Americans understand the potential health dangers associated with excess body weight and few enjoy being fat, a very small proportion actually succeed in achieving permanent weight loss. Instead, most adopt what noted nutritionist Jean Mayer calls "the rhythm method of girth control"; the cycle looks something like this:

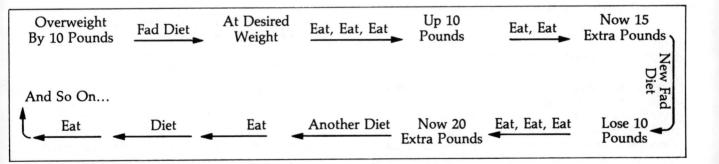

Weight may appear stable according to the scales, while the body can actually be growing fatter! Most dieters step on the scales with fear, yet with complete faith in its reflections. Unfortunately, scales are an unreliable indicator of the true amount of body fat, because how much the body weighs differs from the degree of fatness. Bone and muscle weigh more than fat, and body fluids weigh about the same. Thus, body weight in excess of a given standard does not indicate how much of the extra is from body fat.

There is another reason that scales cannot serve as a reliable gauge of fatness: human weight is extremely variable. Body weight fluctuates continuously during the day due to the on-going accumulation and loss of body fluids. From the following list, check (✔) those factors which could have an effect on your weight—according to the scales, that is:

____ food in digestive tract
____ fluids consumed during the day
____ total salt content of recent dietary intake
____ amount of recent physical activity
____ weather (including degree of humidity)
____ medicinal usage
____ digestive capabilities (including occurrence of constipation or diarrhea)
____ menstrual cycle

When you step on the scales, that weight which is reflected is affected by all of the above factors; the contents of your digestive tract and the level of fluids in your body are influenced by these factors and—in conjunction with the degree of accuracy of the scales themselves—will determine your scale weight. It is best to weigh yourself before breakfast on well-balanced doctor's scales. Yet, keep in mind the idea that, because body weight is so variable, the scales can only serve as a guide.

STEP 3: CALORIES DEFINED

Most overweight Americans are quite concerned about their excess poundage, and are constantly trying to dispose of it through a wide variety of methods. Most of these weight loss schemes are unsuccessful, however, because dieters usually have false concepts of how and why the body gains and loses fat. Overweight people need not feel gluttonous since, in most cases, they are merely the victims of family destiny and the powerful physiological and psychological forces of modern society. Yet, all of these factors can be kept in balance—all that is required is some nutrition know-how and

calorie common sense. There is no need to undertake those costly, dangerous, typically unsuccessful fad diets, crash programs, and quick weight loss schemes (more about these on Day Sixteen). Instead, weight can be kept under control, successfully and permanently, through calorie common sense—an understanding of how food provides energy and of how the body uses this energy.

In terms of body energy, the unit of measurement is the calorie. Foods do not contain calories, as they contain nutrients. Rather, foods provide us with energy, which we measure in calories.

Decide if each of the following statements is True or False:

____ A food might be high in energy value, yet low in caloric content.
____ Vitamins do not provide calories.
____ Vitamins do supply energy.

If a food has few calories, then it provides us with little energy. A food high in caloric content, however, serves as a good source of energy. Vitamins do not provide us with calories. Adequate vitamin intake assists in the maintenance of health and, although good health may make us feel more energetic, true body energy is only provided by calorie-containing foodstuffs.

Note: The term "calorie" is used to describe the energy potential of foods. However, energy is actually measured in "kilocalories" (1000 calories), so the more accurate term is kilocalorie. But since calories are too small to use conveniently (eg, an apple would have 60,000 calories vs 60 kilocalories), and the term kilocalorie is too long to use conveniently, we measure in kilocalories yet talk in calories.

STEP 4: FORMULA FOR CALORIE CONTROL

The basic formulas for determination of weight gain and loss are as follows:

Energy Intake > Energy Expenditure → Weight Gain
Energy Intake < Energy Expenditure → Weight Loss
Energy Intake = Energy Expenditure → Weight Maintenance

Energy is never lost, but is used by or stored in the body. If we take in more energy than we use, the extra is stored as body fat. To get rid of the energy stores, an energy deficit must be created; when energy intake is appropriately low, the body then turns to its fat stores for energy.

In terms of calories, the formulas for weight gain/weight loss are the same:

> Calories Provided (by food) > Calories Used (by bodily function and physical activity) → Weight Gain
> Calories Provided < Calories Used → Weight Loss
> Calories Provided = Calories Used → Weight Maintenance

Thus, beware of diet claims which promise weight loss along with unrestricted caloric intake. Such diets usually result only in loss of body fluids, not body fat. To dispose of body fat stores, more calories must be used than are provided by the diet.

In numerical terms, the key number is 3500. Approximately 3500 calories of energy are furnished by one pound of body fat. It takes an excess of 3500 calories to create a pound of body fat and a deficit of 3500 calories to get rid of a pound of body fat.

Which of the following selections would, if eaten in addition to the required caloric intake, result in the gain of a pound of body fat?

_____ 4 loaves of bread
_____ 12 pounds of baked potatoes
_____ 350 brownies
_____ 1 large chocolate cake, iced
_____ 2 medium pizzas

Each of the above selections provides approximately 3500 calories. Does it seem like a lot of food for a day's intake? Well, in order to lose one pound of body fat in a single day, 3500 calories would have to be used. This would entail, for a healthy 125 pound adult female, the following schedule:

- Diet—water and calorie-free beverages only
- Exercise (to use up 3500 calories)—jogging for about 4 hours, or walking at 3 mph for about 10 hours.

Obviously, it is difficult to gain or lose a pound of body fat in one day. When body weight declines rapidly, it is usually due to loss of body fluids; an effective and permanent weight loss, however, requires a gradual depletion of body fat stores.

STEP 5: BODY RATES

Your body is constantly at work, performing such involuntary activities as digestion, thought, heartbeat, and respiration. Individual bodies work at different rates, depending on:

- age
- sex
- body size
- physical activity
- personal and genetic factors

Body rates decrease with age after infancy. Males usually have faster body rates than females. Lean people tend to have quicker body rates than their fatter counterparts, and the physically active and/or nervously hyperactive persons have body rates which are more rapid than the sedentary and/or relaxed types.

Energy is required to support the body's work. Unless involved in strenuous physical work or athletic activity, the body rate accounts for most of the energy (calories) we use. Thus, age, sex, body size, physical activity, and personal and genetic factors influence the number of calories an individual requires.

The need for calories gradually declines after the first birthday and, after growth, drops about 10% with each decade. Muscle uses more energy than fat, so most males require more calories than females, and those who are physically in shape need a greater number of calories than their fatter friends. There are also some strong hereditary influences on caloric needs, including the body's facility for fat storage and body composition; individuals with greater fat storage capacities tend to be overweight, as do those with the "endomorph" body composition. The chart on page 58 summarizes somatotypes, or body composition categories. Most people are a combination of types.

Therefore, your age, sex, size, and body composition all affect your body rate and thereby determine your caloric needs. There is little we can do to alter any of these factors. However, we can control our caloric requirements to some degree via physical activity: the more active we are, the more calories we need. Thus, body weight is more easily controlled if a program of regular physical activity is undertaken.

STEP 6: YOUR ACTIVITY LEVEL

The physical activity level typical of most Americans is sedentary or light. For most of us, our lifestyles do not incorporate much daily exercise. We drive or take public transportation to work and on errands; we opt for elevators instead of stairs; we utilize numerous household gadgets to save time (and energy); and we spend far more time in front of the television than at the jogging track. Do you consider your general lifestyle to be:

☐ Sedentary/Light in activity
☐ Moderately active
☐ Physically Strenuous

Somatotype	Physical Description			
	Body Frame	Body Characteristics	Appetite	Activity Level
Endomorph	rounded, pear-shaped figure	pudgy hands and feet, bulky abdomen and hips, great fat storage capacity	no distinct appetite cutoff	inactive, slow, tendency to rest for long intervals
Ectomorph	slight, thin	long thin hands and feet with narrow fingers, wiry muscles, little fat storage capacity	distinct appetite cutoff	active, fidgety
Mesomorph	broad shoulders, heavy bones	blunt hands and fingers, sturdy legs, well-formed muscles, fat storage capacity greater than ectomorph and less than endomorph but evenly distributed	no distinct appetite cutoff	tendency for bursts of activity

Use the following chart as a general guideline for determining your own activity level. Note the word "typical"—this does not include sporadic indulgences.

Activity Level	Typical Activities
Sedentary/Light	sitting, standing, watching television, eating, driving, sewing, ironing, cooking, dusting, washing, shopping, painting, typing, lab work, garage work, golfing, sailing, walking 2 to 3 mph
Moderate	walking 3 to 4 mph, gardening, heavy housework, dancing, tennis, bowling
Strenuous	pick and shovel work, logging, ball games, swimming, climbing, bicycling, skiing, running

Keep in mind, however, the fact that individuals vary in the intensities with which they indulge in activities. Imagine yourself involved in the following activities and select the method of participation for each which best describes your typical degree of intensity:

Activity	Method of Participation
Tennis	Play doubles, let partner do most of the retrieval Play singles, constantly in motion
Golf	Ride in golf cart Caddy own clubs on foot
Walking	Saunter casually, never hurriedly Step briskly at a quick pace (3–4 mph)
Cycling	Ride slowly, coasting often Pedal constantly at a quick pace (12–15 mph)
Dancing	Foxtrot, waltz, etc Squaredance, disco, jitterbug, etc
Skiing	After one run, spend day in lounge Many brisk runs
Swimming	Slow, relaxing float Many brisk laps
Sailing	Let others sail and relax with a beer Constantly in motion, at tiller and sails

STEP 7: YOUR WEIGHT GOAL

What should you weigh? How do you determine your weight goal? Height-weight charts do not account for the wide degree of variation among individuals. Height-weight charts merely depict body weights without consideration of body fat. In fact, these charts are like scales—an inaccurate means for determination of body fatness. Try the following methods for a more accurate estimation of your own level of body fat:

- Pinch-Test—There are certain areas of the body where the thickness of the fat deposits under the skin reflect rather accurately the total amount of fat stored in the body; pinch the skin midway between your shoulder and your elbow—can you pinch an inch? More?
- Mirror Test—This is the most revealing, yet most unpleasant way to determine the need for weight loss; without clothing, look in the mirror for obvious body fat deposits—can you see any? Many?

The simplest method for determining your own weight goal is to use the following mathematical formula:

Males = 106 pounds for the first five feet of height + 6 pounds for each additional inch.
Females = 100 pounds for first five feet of height + 5 pounds for each additional inch.

If your body frame is heavy-boned and large, add an additional 10%.

You may prefer to set your goal by using a specific weight at which you once felt comfortable (eg, weight at age 18, weight at time of marriage, etc). Try to be realistic in your goals, and avoid setting a weight goal that will ultimately result in discouragement and feelings of failure. Instead, set a weight goal that will be practical to attain and will provide physical benefits when maintained.

Remember that it took you a long time to acquire the weight you now carry. You have the rest of your life to attain and maintain your desired weight, one that will support your individual needs and contribute to your health and well-being.

Your Present Weight: _____ pounds
Your Weight Goal: _____ pounds

STEP 8: YOUR CALORIE NEEDS

In order to determine your own caloric requirements, use the following formula:

Your Weight Goal		Your Activity Level Factor		Your Average Daily Caloric
_____ pounds	×	13 (sedentary/light)	=	Need for Maintenance
(see Step 7)		15 (moderate)		_____ calories
		20 (strenuous)		(round to nearest hundredth)
		(see Step 6)		

Your average daily caloric need for maintenance is the approximate number of calories you require to maintain your weight goal.

Next, use the following formula to determine the calorie level which will allot for your desired weekly weight loss:

Your Average Daily Caloric Need for Maintenance	Caloric Decrease (per day)		Your Average Daily Caloric Need		Average No. Pounds to be Lost (per week)
	250	=	_____ calories →		½
	500	=	_____ calories →		1
_____ calories —	750	=	_____ calories →		1½
	1000	=	_____ calories →		2
	1250	=	_____ calories →		2½
	1500	=	_____ calories →		3
	(round to nearest hundredth)				

Using these formulas, you can determine the approximate number of calories you require each day to lose the desired number of pounds per week. In order to simplify the use of these formulas, a sample determination has been illustrated on page 60.

Note: A caloric intake below 1000 for women or 1200 for men is apt to be nutritionally inadequate and only temporary in duration. An important goal for anyone seeking permanent success in weight loss is to avoid quick-loss schemes in preference to a well-balanced diet plan that allots for the safe and effective loss of pounds at a gradual rate.

STEP 9: CALORIE COUNTING

How many daily calories do you usually take in? Use your Nutri-Plan diet diary and a calorie chart to determine the number of calories you obtained from your dietary intake on Day One. In the chart on page 61, list all foods and beverages consumed on Day One and the amounts. Then determine the number of calories per serving. Total your caloric intake for Day One. Compare this total to your average daily caloric need which you determined in Step 8. Are these numbers similar, or did you take in more/less calories than you need?

Repeat this procedure to estimate your caloric intake on Day Eight. Does your caloric intake appear to be increasing or decreasing? To what can you attribute any changes?

Note: "Total calories" is merely an estimate, since the true caloric content varies widely from food to food (eg, an apple may be 50 calories or it may be 110, depending on variety, season, exact size, etc), and actual caloric absorption may differ as well.

STEP 10: DAY NINE PLAN

Continue to record everything you eat and drink in your Nutri-Plan diet diary. For Day Nine, continue to be aware of your intake of protein, carbohydrate, fat, vitamins, minerals and water. Also, pay careful attention to the types of foods you are eating in order that you may include the recommended number of servings from the basic food groups; watch out for an excessive dependence on foods from the Others Group.

At the end of Day Nine, complete another chart totaling your caloric intake, using the methods you utilized in Step 9. Note also the corresponding basic food groups for each food and beverage consumed. How closely did you approximate your average daily caloric need? Did you include the recommended number of servings from each basic food group? How many selections from the Others Group did you consume, and did these selections

Sample

1) Your Weight Goal   ×   Your Activity Level Factor   =   Your Average Daily
    135 pounds   ⑬ (sedentary/light)   Caloric Need
                                     15 (moderate)   for Maintenance
                                     20 (strenuous)   *1755* calories

2) Your Average Daily   ──▶ (round to nearest hundredth) =   Your Average Daily
    Caloric Need   Caloric Need
    for Maintenance   for Maintenance
    1755 calories   *1800* calories

3) Your Average Daily   Caloric Decrease   Your Average Daily   Average No. Pounds
    Caloric Need   (per day)   Caloric Need   To Lose ──▶   to be Lost
    for Maintenance   (per week)

    1800 calories   —   250   =   _____   ½
                                    500   1
                                   ⟨750⟩   *1050*   ⟨1½⟩
                                   1000   _____   2
                                   1250   _____   2½
                                   1500   _____   3

4) In desiring an average number pounds to be lost (per week) of 1½ pounds, your average daily caloric need is 1050 calories. Again, round to the nearest hundredth: 1100 calories.

Sample Results

Your Weight Goal	Average Daily Caloric Needs	Average No. Pounds to be Lost (per week)
135 pounds	*1100* calories	*1½* pounds

Your Average Daily Caloric Need

1) Your Weight Goal   ×   Your Activity Level Factor   =   Your Average Daily
    _____ pounds   13 (sedentary/light)   Caloric Need
                                     15 (moderate)   for Maintenance
                                     20 (strenuous)   _____ calories

2) Your Average Daily   ──▶ (round to nearest hundredth) =   Your Average Daily
    Caloric Need   Caloric Need
    for Maintenance   for Maintenance
    _____ calories   _____ calories

3) Your Average Daily   Caloric Decrease   Your Average Daily   Average No. Pounds
    Caloric Need   (per day)   Caloric Need   To Lose ──▶   to be Lost
    for Maintenance   (per week)

    _____ calories —   250   =   _____   ½
                                    500   _____   1
                                    750   _____   1½
                                   1000   _____   2
                                   1250   _____   2½
                                   1500   _____   3

4) In desiring an average number pounds to be lost (per week) of _____ pounds, your average daily caloric need is _____ calories. Again, round to the nearest hundredth: _____ calories.

Your Results

Your Weight Goal	Average Daily Caloric Needs	Average No. Pounds to be Lost (per week)
_____ pounds	_____ calories	_____ pounds

Day One

Food and Amount	Calories

Total Calories: _____ Calories
Your Average Daily Caloric Need: _____ Calories

Day Eight

Food and Amount	Calories

Total Calories: _____ Calories
Your Average Daily Caloric Need: _____ Calories

tend to be higher in calories than your other dietary choices?

Might it not prove easier overall to plan ahead? By mapping out your intended day's intake, you may be able to ensure that you remain within a desirable caloric range, yet obtain your nutrient needs. A diet planned in advance can help you to avoid the exclusion of necessary foods, while assisting you to minimize your intake of less desirable foodstuffs. Diet planning is an integral aspect of balancing the diet, and some of the practical steps involved will be explained in detail on Day Twenty-Two.

STEP 1: WHO IS GEORGE?

Although some important factors which influence health are not under our own control (eg, heredity and accidents), there also exists a large number of choices we can make in order to determine our states of physical well-being. Consider the following statements carefully before checking (✔) the answers which best describe your personal habits:

Yes No
☐ ☐ I smoke cigarettes.
☐ ☐ I sometimes drink alcohol excessively.
☐ ☐ I do not exercise regularly.
☐ ☐ I am overweight.
☐ ☐ My diet is not well balanced.

The above statements concern five factors which directly influence health and well-being. The choices—to not smoke, to be moderate in alcohol consumption, to exercise on a regular basis, to maintain desirable weight, and to eat well—are all your own. You have already chosen to moderate your dietary intake. In so doing, you may also find that you are making other changes in the pursuit of good health; you might:

• Lose some weight.
• Adopt a program of regular exercise.
• Cut down on alcohol intake.
• Stop smoking.

According to the former senator from South Dakota, George McGovern, and the US Senate's special Select Committee on Nutrition and Human Needs,

> "The simple fact is that our diets have changed radically within the past fifty years, with great and often very harmful effects on our health... In all, six of the ten leading causes of death in the United States have been linked with our diet."

In 1977 and 1978, this Committee, led by Senator George McGovern, published two editions of *Dietary Goals* intended for the American public. *Dietary Goals* recommended certain changes in diet in order to reduce our risks for developing cancer, heart disease, stroke, obesity, chronic liver disease, and other related degenerative diseases.

The goals were effective in that they generated widespread publicity. Newspapers, radio, television, and magazines all informed the public about the suggested dietary goals and their possible effects on health. The various controversies which surrounded these recommendations by the Senate committee served only to add to the publicity given to the current American diet and the need for change. *Dietary Goals*, however, was never endorsed by government agencies and is not legislation. Actually, *Dietary Goals* is no more than a staff report, written by legislative assistants as an interpretation of the advice of selected professionals.

In February of 1980, the US Department of Agriculture and the US Department of Health, Education, and Welfare released a very similar report entitled *Nutrition and Your Health— Dietary Guidelines for Americans*. Disappointingly enough, it generated little media reaction. The *Dietary Guidelines* appear to be a simplified version of the *Dietary Goals* and include the following sensible suggestions:

• Eat a variety of foods.
• Maintain ideal weight.
• Avoid too much fat, saturated fat, and cholesterol.
• Eat foods with adequate starch and fiber.
• Avoid too much sugar.
• Avoid too much sodium.
• If you drink alcohol, do so in moderation.

National dietary policy appears to be of questionable popularity and of doubtful probability in

63

the near future. It is up to you to look for the facts, weigh the information, and make your own decisions concerning nutrition and your diet.

STEP 2: WHAT ARE THE GOALS?

The US Senate Select Committee on Nutrition and Human Needs suggested that Americans should decrease the consumption of certain foods and increase the intake of others. The second and most recent edition of the *Goals*, released in February of 1978, recommended that we make the following dietary changes:

• Increase the consumption of complex carbohydrates and naturally occurring sugars from 28% of energy intake to about 48% of total energy intake.
• Reduce the consumption of refined and other processed sugars by about 48%.
• Reduce overall fat consumption from about 40% to about 30% of total energy intake.
• Reduce saturated fat consumption to about 10% of total energy intake, and balance that with polyunsaturated and monounsaturated fats, each accounting for 10% of total energy intake.
• Reduce cholesterol consumption to about 300 mg daily.
• Reduce salt intake to about five grams* per day.

The *Goals* also suggested that, in order to avoid overweight, we should consume only as much energy as we expend, and if overweight, we should reduce energy intake and increase energy expenditure.

All these numbers and percentages make use of the *Goals* impractical for everyday menu planning. A simplified version of the *Goals* can provide you with a more general yet clearer understanding of the suggested changes:

• Increase consumption of fruits, vegetables, and whole grains.
• Reduce consumption of meat, and increase consumption of poultry and fish.
• Reduce intake of high-fat foods (whole milk, cream, butter, fried foods, fatty meats), and partially substitute polyunsaturated fats (vegetable oils, salad dressings, margarine) for saturated fats (hydrogenated fats, coconut and palm oil, butter).
• Reduce consumption of butter, eggs, organ meats, and other high-cholesterol foods.
• Reduce consumption of sugar and foods high in sugar content (soft drinks, pastries, presweetened cereals, candy, desserts, sweets).
• Reduce consumption of salt and foods high in

---

*Note: Refers only to added salt; total daily sodium intake should be around 8 grams.

salt content (pickles, chips, crackers, condiments, soups).

Have you made any of the above changes in your diet during the past nine days? Use your Nutri-Plan diet diary and the simplified list of the *Dietary Goals* to carefully consider and answer the following questions:

1) Which of the dietary goals have you already begun working toward?
_____

2) Cite some examples of dietary changes made since Day One that are in accordance with the goals (eg, switched to margarine from butter):
_____

3) Which of the dietary goals do you intend to adopt in the future?
_____

4) Give some examples of how you plan to change your diet in order to adopt these goals (eg, cook with vegetable oils rather than butter):
_____
_____

Deeper evaluation of these dietary changes will be possible during the next six days, while you learn how easy it is to eat for good health!

STEP 3: HEALTHY PEOPLE

In July of 1979, the *US Surgeon General's Report on Health Promotion and Disease Prevention* was released after over two years of preparation by the Department of Health, Education, and Welfare and one of their branches, the Surgeon General's Office. This 150 page document is called *Healthy People,* and it elaborates on the suggestions of the *Dietary Goals. Healthy People* suggests that we adopt the following lifestyle changes:

• Avoid cigarette smoking.
• Eat more nutritious foods.
• Drink less alcohol.
• Get more physical exercise.
• Obtain adequate prenatal care.
• Strive to create an environment which is more conducive to health and energy.

The report includes recommendations concerning a variety of health issues, ranging from breastfeeding and home safety to mental health care and medical exams. *Healthy People* suggests five goals for America to strive toward during the 1980s:

• Improve infant health so that infant mortality is reduced by at least 35%.
• Improve child health and reduce deaths among children aged 1 to 14 by at least 20%.

- Improve teen health habits to reduce deaths among those aged 15 to 24 by at least 20%.
- Improve adult health and reduce deaths among those aged 25 to 64 by at least 25%.
- Improve health and quality of life for the elderly and reduce the average annual number of days of restricted activity due to acute and chronic conditions by 20%.

From prenatal to the elderly years, diet can play an integral role in the achievement of such goals. The dietary modifications suggested by *Healthy People*, quite similar to those made by the *Dietary Goals* and *Dietary Guidelines* include the following:

- more complex carbohydrates such as fruits, vegetables, and whole grains
- less red meat, and more fish and poultry
- less saturated fat
- less cholesterol
- less sugar
- less salt
- adequate calories to attain and maintain desirable body weight

Healthy People, the *Dietary Guidelines*, and the *Dietary Goals* are controversial reports, and their recommendations serve as an ongoing subject for heated debate among the medical profession, government, food industries, consumer activists, nutritionists, scientists, and the public.

In order to avoid total confusion—or blind devotion to any one school of thought—you may want to read the reports for yourself; you can send for them at the addresses given in the Recommended References (Appendix C). And in making your own evaluations, consider the following concepts:

- Scientific documentation is different from hopes and beliefs.
- Research results can be interpreted differently, depending on the interests of the interpreter.
- In scientific research, nothing is proven; evidence can merely indicate.
- Science is always advancing, so our nutrition concepts must grow and develop concurrently.

STEP 4: YOUR GOALS FOR HEALTH

Is your diet a healthy one? Does it incorporate the suggestions provided by the *Dietary Goals? Dietary Guidelines? Healthy People?* Use your Nutri-Plan diet diary to determine whether your diet incorporated these recommendations on Day One. In the chart on page 66, list all food and beverages consumed on Day One and the amounts. Then answer the associated questions. Was your diet on Day One "health-promoting" in its make-up? Repeat this procedure to examine your dietary intake for Day Nine. In accordance with the *Dietary Goals*, *Dietary Guidelines*, and *Healthy People*, did you make any desirable dietary changes? Can you see any aspects of your diet that you want to change in the future?

Note that dietary suggestions of the *Dietary Goals*, the *Dietary Guidelines*, and *Healthy People* are intended for normal, healthy adults. The dietary needs of infants, children, and persons who are elderly, pregnant, or ill require special individual consideration.

STEP 5: DAY TEN PLAN

Continue to record everything you eat and drink in your Nutri-Plan diet diary. For Day Ten, continue to be aware of your intake of protein, carbohydrate, fat, vitamins, minerals, and water. Also pay careful attention to the types of foods you are eating in order that you may include the recommended number of servings from the basic food groups; watch out for an excessive dependence on foods from the Others Group.

At the end of Day Ten, complete another chart totaling your caloric intake using the methods you utilized on Day Nine. Compare the total to your average daily caloric need. Then repeat the questionnaire from Step 4 of Day Ten. Do you notice any changes from Day One to Day Nine to Day Ten?

As a matter of fact, during the past ten days you have probably already begun to incorporate some of the suggestions of the *Dietary Goals*, *Dietary Guidelines*, and *Healthy People* into your own diet. Successful dietary change is simply a matter of acquiring nutrition education and making wise food selections. You are on your way!

66

Day One

Food and Amount

Day Nine

Food and Amount

Associated Questions

Day One
Yes No

Day Nine
Yes No

1) Did you have two or more servings of fruit?

2) Did you have two or more servings of vegetables?

3) Did you have four or more servings of whole grain products?

4) Did you select poultry or fish in preference to red meat?

5) Did you include any of the following high-fat foods: butter, cream, whole milk, whole milk cheeses, fatty meats, ice cream, fried foods, nuts, coconut oil, palm oil, lard?

6) Did you include any of the following high-cholesterol foods: egg yolk, organ meats, fatty meats, shrimp, butter, cream, whole milk, whole milk cheeses?

7) Did you include any of the following high-sugar foods: donuts, pastries, sweet desserts, candy, presweetened cereals, jams, jellies, honey, syrups, sugars, soft drinks, chewing gum?

8) Did you include any of the following high-salt foods: smoked/dried meat or fish, canned fish, bacon, luncheon meats, salted nuts, pickled vegetables, sauerkraut, crackers, olives, condiments, chips, soups, seasoned salts, table salt?

9) Did you take in more calories than you need? (See Day Nine for your average daily caloric need.)

DAY ELEVEN

FRUIT AND VEGETABLE GROUP

STEP 1: COMPARING CHOICES

One of the dietary changes suggested by the *Dietary Goals*, *Dietary Guidelines*, and *Healthy People* is an increased consumption of fruits and vegetables. The basic food groups can guide in the selection of four or more daily servings. Unfortunately, most Americans tend not to consume enough fruits and vegetables, succumbing instead to tempting selections from the Others Group.

In the list below, circle the food from each pair that you would be most likely to choose for a typical snack or as part of an average meal. The correct or wisest answer may seem obvious in some instances, but try to make your selections as honestly as possible—the wisest answers are usually not the most popular!

- fresh blackberries or blackberry pie
- sliced banana or banana split
- pineapple chunks or pineapple upside-down cake
- fresh strawberries or strawberry shortcake
- fresh orange juice or orange-flavored drink
- fresh peach slices or peach ice cream
- tossed salad or tossed salad with blue cheese dressing
- boiled cabbage or coleslaw
- broiled mushrooms or deep fried mushrooms
- steamed broccoli or French fried onion rings
- raw carrot sticks or carrot cake

Now compare the nutritional and caloric values for each of the selections in the pairs listed above (see chart on page 70). Perhaps the results will influence your food choices. It is simply a matter of nutritional priorities.

Fruits and vegetables are largely composed of carbohydrate, so are naturally low in calories. But when fat is added during preparation, caloric contents are notably increased. (Remember that fat provides more than twice as many calories per gram or per ounce as carbohydrate.) And although the addition of sugar does not increase caloric contents as much as the addition of fat, the sugar calories are not accompanied by vitamins and minerals—nor fiber, for that matter. Thus, sweetened fruit products have extra calories, but lack nutrient enhancement; in fact, processing may result in some nutrient and fiber losses.

Obviously, the fresher and plainer the produce, the better it is for you—nutritionally and calorically. When the choice is yours, why not opt for the low-calorie, vitamin-rich, mineral-rich, fibrous produce selections?

STEP 2: AND FIBER, FOR THAT MATTER

Not only is it important to include carbohydrate in the diet, but it is essential to consume the best types of carbohydrate. Fruits and vegetables can serve as good sources of the desirable types of carbohydrate. All types of produce can provide carbohydrate accompanied by various vitamins and minerals, since the starches and sugars present in these plant foods are naturally nutrient-rich.

Fruits and vegetables also contain considerable amounts of fiber. Fiber is the portion of carbohydrate which humans are unable to digest completely. Dr. John Harvey Kellogg of cereal fame coined the term "nature's broom," which gives a

Food and Amount	Calories	High In:
blackberries, fresh, 1 cup	84	fiber, vitamin C, potassium
blackberry pie, 3½" arc	287	sugar, fat
banana, small	81	fiber, potassium
banana split, average size	785	sugar, fat
pineapple chunks, unsweetened, 1 cup	96	fiber, vitamin C, potassium
pineapple upside-down cake, 3" arc	270	sugar, fat
strawberries, fresh, 1 cup	55	fiber, vitamin C, potassium
strawberry shortcake, large biscuit	420	sugar, fat
orange juice, unsweetened, 1 cup	112	vitamin C, potassium
orange fruit-flavored drink, 1 cup	130	sugar (may be vitamin C-fortified)
peach slices, fresh, 1 cup	65	fiber, vitamin A, potassium
peach ice cream, 1 cup	330	sugar, fat, calories, riboflavin
tossed salad (lettuce, cucumber, tomato, sprouts), 1 cup	35	fiber, vitamin A, folic acid, potassium
tossed salad with blue cheese dressing, 1 tbsp	111	fat, fiber, vitamin A, folic acid, potassium
cabbage, boiled, 1 cup	31	fiber, vitamin C
coleslaw, 1 cup	173	fat, fiber, vitamin C
mushrooms, broiled, ½ cup	50	fiber, potassium
mushrooms, deep fried, large serving	300	fat, sodium (salt)
broccoli, steamed, 1 cup	40	fiber, vitamin A, vitamin C, calcium, magnesium
French fried onion rings, large serving	330	fat, sodium (salt)
carrot sticks, raw, 6 to 8 (1 oz)	12	fiber, vitamin A
carrot cake, average slice	380	sugar, fat

vivid picture of fibrous foods sweeping through the intestinal tract. This process is beneficial to the overall health of the digestive system, and adequate fiber in the diet will:

- increase bulk so that larger, softer stools are produced on a more frequent basis.
- decrease the amount of time undigested food spends in the intestines.
- decrease straining with elimination.

The possible health benefits associated with these changes include:

- alleviation and prevention of constipation.
- decreased incidence of intestinal disease including diverticular diseases, appendicitis, irritable bowel syndrome, and cancer of the colon.

An increase in dietary fiber has also been suggested as one part of the treatment of diabetes, obesity, and coronary heart disease.

The beneficial effects of dietary fiber in the prevention and cure of all of the above disorders, however, requires further research and documentation. And as commonly occurs with all health discoveries, the food faddists have joined in the fiber fury with exaggerated claims, undocumented research results, and excessively costly high-fiber products.

Although the optimal dietary amount has not yet been established, it is believed that Americans do need an increased fiber intake. Yet, most Americans are perpetuating the current trend toward a decreased intake.

Usually, the more a product has been refined and

processed, the less total dietary fiber it contains. This is illustrated by the refining process of whole grains (described in detail on Day Twelve), and should also be a consideration in the selection of fruits and vegetables:

- Juice has less fiber than the fruit or vegetable from which it is derived.
- Skins and seeds add to the fiber content of produce.
- Raw fruits and vegetables do contain somewhat more fiber than their cooked counterparts, and the less cooking time the better.

In the list below, circle the product in each pair which you think probably contains the most fiber:

- Fresh apple or applesauce
- Sliced peaches or peach nectar
- Spinach salad or creamed spinach
- Tomato slices or tomato sauce
- Steamed asparagus or cream of asparagus soup
- Dried apricots or apricot jelly

The first choice in each pair tends to be less refined and is a richer source of fiber.

The chart below shows the fiber contents of several common foods:

Food and Amount	Dietary Fiber in grams per 100 grams of food	Crude Fiber in grams per 100 grams of food
apples, without skin	1.42	.6
lettuce, raw	1.53	.6
strawberries, raw	2.12	1.3
peaches, with skin	2.28	.6
white bread	2.72	.2
carrots, boiled	3.70	1.0
broccoli tops, boiled	4.10	1.5
sweet corn, cooked	4.74	.7
peas, canned	6.28	2.3
peanut butter	7.55	1.9
Brazil nuts	7.73	3.1
whole wheat bread	8.50	1.6
peanuts	9.30	1.9
cornflakes	11.0	.7
All-bran cereal	26.7	7.8

Note that the dietary fiber content of foods differs from the crude fiber content. Crude fiber is the undissolved plant material remaining after prolonged treatment with acid and alkali; dietary fiber is that portion of plants thought not to be digestible by the human digestive tract. Thus, dietary fiber is not interchangeable with crude fiber; values for dietary fiber are usually higher, because our digestive system is appreciably less efficient than the chemical treatment used to determine crude fiber. Keep in mind that, as is common with food composition tables, the data on fiber are merely estimates and should be used for general informational purposes only.

STEP 3: LET'S LIST THEM

In the chart on page 72, list as many different types of fruits as you can think of. Check (✓) those fruits which you have never eaten, those you tend to avoid, and those fruits which you do include in your diet.

Next repeat the above identification process in the vegetable chart on page 73.

Note: The following vegetables are higher than most in starch and calories, so since they are nutritionally comparable to grains, they are included in the Grain Group rather than the Fruit and Vegetable Group:

- corn
- dried beans and peas, lentils
- parsnips
- peas
- potato, sweet potato
- pumpkin
- winter squash
- yam

Next, compare your fruit list to the one given below, and your vegetable list to the one that follows. You may find that you have never even heard of some of these foods! Actually, fruits and vegetables are a lot less dull than you may think. Creative imagination and the courage to try new foods can expose you to all sorts of new taste sensations. A variety of delicious and nutritious produce recipes are given on Days Twenty-One and Twenty-Three.

Fruit List		
Acerola cherries	Grapefruit	Persimmon
Apple	Grapes	Pineapple
Apricots, dried	Ground cherries	Plantain
Apricots, fresh	Guava	Plums
Banana	Honeydew melon	Pomegranate
Blackberries	Kiwi	Prunes
Blueberries	Kumquat	Quince
Boysenberries	Logenberries	Raisins
Cantaloupe	Mango	Raspberries
Casaba melon	Orange	Strawberries
Cherries	Papaw	Tangelo
Cranberries	Papaya	Tangerine
Currants	Passion fruit	Watermelon
Dates	Peach	
Figs	Pear	

Fruit	Never Eaten (✔)	Tend to Avoid (✔)	Do Eat (✔)

Vegetable List

Alfalfa sprouts	Chinese cabbage	Squash, summer
Artichoke	Cilantro	(patty pan, scallop,
Asparagus	Cucumber	summer, zucchini)
Bamboo shoots	Eggplant	Tomatoes
Bean sprouts	Kohlrabi	Turnip
Beans, green	Lettuce	Water chestnuts
Beans, wax	Mushrooms	
Beets	Okra	
Broccoli	Onions	
Brussels sprouts	Pepper, green	
Cabbage	Pepper, red	
Carrots	Radishes	
Cauliflower	Rhubarb	
Celery	Rutabaga	
Chayote	Sauerkraut	
Chicory	Snow peas	

Greens (beet, collard, dandelion, endive, garden
  cress, kale, mustard, parsley, spinach,
  Swiss chard, turnip, watercress)

STEP 4: IDENTIFYING NUTRIENTS

Although the Fruit and Vegetable Group is noted as rich in vitamins and minerals, only certain items contain appreciable amounts of the various nutrients. You may want to use the charts on page 74 in order to assist you in the selection of those produce items which are abundant in specific vitamins and/or minerals.

Remember that most fruits and vegetables do contain differing amounts of a variety of vitamins and minerals, plus fiber. A diet which includes a variety of fruits and vegetables can help to ensure the intake of the many different nutrients needed by the body.

STEP 5: FRUITS AND VEGETABLES IN YOUR DIET

Do you think that you include the recommended number of fruit and vegetable servings in your

Vegetable	Never Eaten (✔)	Tend to Avoid (✔)	Do Eat (✔)

daily diet? Are your produce choices especially high in vitamins, minerals, and/or fiber? Use your Nutri-Plan diet diary to determine whether your diet included the proper number of recommended servings from the Fruit and Vegetable Group on Day Ten. Then, using the charts in this chapter, check to see if your selections were those richest in fiber, vitamins, and/or minerals. In the chart on page 75, list all fruits and vegetables (and their juices) consumed on Day Ten, and total the number of servings. Check (✔) any accompanying nutrients. Also note the following:

• Were most of your fruit and vegetable choices eaten raw?
• Did you eat the skins and/or seeds?
• Did you select the whole fruit or vegetable in preference to the juice?
• Did you tend to choose plain fruits and vegetables instead of the more sugary, fatty versions?

Remember that the fruit and vegetable contents of your diet, when selected and prepared wisely, can donate essential nutrients and fiber.

STEP 6: DAY ELEVEN PLAN

Continue to record everything you eat and drink in your Nutri-Plan diet diary. For Day Eleven, continue to be aware of your intake of protein, carbohydrate, fat, vitamins, minerals, and water. Try to approximate your personal needs, and to select foods wisely from the basic food groups; watch out for an excessive dependence on foods from the Others Group.

On Day Eleven, eat a fruit and/or vegetable which you have never eaten before. Eat it raw, with the skin and seeds if possible, or cook it lightly. Then complete the fruit and vegetable questionnaire on the next page. Remember that fruits and vegetables, when selected and prepared with nutrition know-how, can add considerable nutrients and fiber to your diet. And they can be as delicious as they are nutritious.

Rich in Vitamin C		Rich in Vitamin A	
acerola cherries	broccoli	apricots	asparagus
blackberries	Brussels sprouts	cantaloupe	broccoli
cantaloupe	cabbage	ground cherries	carrots
grapefruit	cauliflower	mango	green leafy vegetables:
guava	green leafy vegetables:	papaya	beet greens
honeydew melon	collard greens	peach	collard greens
loganberries	garden cress	persimmons	dandelion greens
mango	kale	pokeberries	endive
oranges	mustard greens	prunes	kale
papaya	parsley		mustard greens
pineapple	spinach		parsley
pokeberries	turnip		spinach
strawberries	watercress		Swiss chard
tangelo	kohlrabi		turnip greens
tangerine	okra		watercress
	pepper, green		okra
	pepper, red		pepper, red
	potato*		rhubarb
	radishes		squash, winter*
	rutabaga		tomato
	sauerkraut		
	squash, winter*		
	sweet potato*		
	turnip		

Rich in Calcium	Rich in Iron	
green leafy vegetables:	dates	asparagus
collard greens	pokeberries	Brussels sprouts
kale	prunes	green leafy vegetables:
mustard greens	raisins	beet greens
turnip greens	raspberries	collard greens
		dandelion greens
Rich in Folic Acid		kale
		mustard greens
asparagus		parsley
bean sprouts		spinach
green leafy vegetables:		Swiss chard
collard greens		turnip greens
endive		rhubarb
kale		squash, winter*
spinach		
Swiss chard		
turnip greens		

*Actually considered as Grain Group servings rather than vegetables.

Fruit and Vegetable Questionnaire

1) What new fruit and/or vegetable did you include in your diet on Day Eleven?_____

2) Was it eaten raw?_____ Lightly cooked_____ If cooked, describe type of preparation (eg, steamed, stir-fried, etc): _____

3) Did you eat the skin?_____ Seeds?_____

4) Did you like this new food?_____ Why or why not? _____

5) Please add any additional comments you may want to make:_____
   _____

Day Ten

Fruit/Vegetable and Amount	Rich in (✔)					
	Fiber	Vitamin A	Vitamin C	Calcium	Iron	Folic Acid

Total fruit and vegetable servings:_____
No. of recommended servings: 4 or more

DAY TWELVE

GRAIN GROUP

STEP 1: COMPARING CHOICES

One of the dietary changes suggested by the *Dietary Goals, Dietary Guidelines*, and *Healthy People* is an increased consumption of whole grain products. The basic food groups can guide us in the selection of four or more daily servings. Unfortunately, most Americans tend not to consume enough whole grain foods, succumbing instead to tempting selections from the Others Group.

In the list below, circle the food from each pair that you would be most likely to choose for a typical snack or as part of an average meal. The correct or wisest answer may seem obvious in some instances, but try to make your selections as honestly as possible—the wisest answers are usually not the most popular!

- shredded wheat cereal or granola bar
- buckwheat pancakes or blueberry pancakes
- whole rye toast or English muffin with jam
- oatmeal with raisins or sugared donut
- whole wheat crackers or soda crackers
- cornbread or banana bread
- pumpernickel bagel or Danish pastry
- whole wheat bread or white bread
- brown rice or white rice
- whole wheat spaghetti or egg noodles

Now compare the nutritional and caloric values for each of the selections in the pairs listed above (see chart on page 78). Perhaps the results will influence your food choices. It is simply a matter of nutritional priorities.

Whole grains are largely composed of carbohydrate, so are naturally low in calories. But when fat is added during preparation, caloric content are noticeably increased. (Remember that fat provides more than twice as many calories per gram or per ounce as carbohydrate). And although the addition of sugar does not increase the caloric content as much as the addition of fat, the sugar calories are not accompanied by vitamins and minerals—nor by fiber, for that matter. Thus, sweetened grain products have extra calories, but lack nutrient enhancement; in fact, processing may result in some nutrient and fiber losses.

Obviously, the less processed and plainer the grain product, the better it is for you—nutritionally and calorically. When the choice is yours, why not opt for the low-calorie, vitamin-rich, mineral-rich, fibrous whole grains?

STEP 2: AND FIBER, FOR THAT MATTER

Not only is it important to include carbohydrate in the diet, but it is essential to consume the best types of carbohydrate. Whole grain products can serve as good sources of the desirable types of carbohydrate. Unprocessed or lightly processed grains provide carbohydrate accompanied by various vitamins and minerals because the starch present in grains is naturally nutrient-rich.

Whole grain products also contain considerable amounts of fiber. Remember Dr John Harvey Kellogg's descriptive term "nature's broom" in visualizing fibrous foods sweeping through the intestinal tract, a process of considerable benefit to the health of the digestive system. The exact role of fiber in the prevention of certain diseases is under research.

Food and Amount	Calories	*High In:
shredded wheat, 1 biscuit	89	fiber, B-vitamins, iron, phosphorus, magnesium
granola bar	120	sugar, fat, fiber
buckwheat pancakes, 4″ dia, 2	108	fiber, B-vitamins, iron, phosphorus, magnesium
blueberry pancakes (enriched flour, sweetened berries), 4″ dia, 2	152	sugar
whole rye bread	61	fiber, B-vitamins, iron, phosphorus, magnesium
English muffin, 1 + strawberry jam, 1 tbsp	70 + 54 = 124	sugar
oatmeal, ¾ cup + raisins, 1 tbsp	99 + 26 = 125	fiber, B-vitamins, iron, phosphorus, potassium, magnesium
sugared donut	233	sugar, fat
whole wheat crackers, unsalted, 2	24	fiber, B-vitamins, iron, phosphorus, magnesium
soda crackers, 2	25	sodium (salt)
cornbread, 2½″ sq	178	fiber, B-vitamins
banana bread, ¾″ slice	150	sugar, fat
pumpernickel bagel	160	fiber, B-vitamins, iron, phosphorus, magnesium
Danish pastry	274	sugar, fat
whole wheat bread	61	fiber, B-vitamins, iron, phosphorus, magnesium
white bread, enriched	63	B-vitamins and iron (replaced with enrichment)
brown rice, ½ cup	116	fiber, B-vitamins, iron, phosphorus, magnesium
white rice, enriched, ½ cup	112	B-vitamins, and iron (replaced with enrichment)
whole wheat spaghetti, 1 cup	195	fiber, B-vitamins, iron, phosphorus, magnesium
egg noodles, enriched, 1 cup	200	B-vitamins and iron (replaced with enrichment)

*Note: Iron is not well absorbed from whole grains because it is bound up by the phytic acid present in whole grain products.

Although the optimal dietary amount has yet to be established, Americans do need an increased fiber intake, yet have been continuing the current trend toward decreased intake.

Usually, the more the product has been refined and processed, the less total dietary fiber it contains. This can be illustrated using the refining of whole grains as an example:

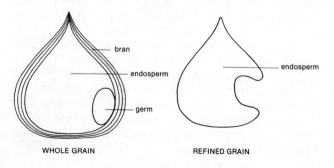

A whole grain is composed of three major components: the outermost layers of bran, the core germ, and the largest portion, endosperm. During milling or refinement, the coarse bran layers are removed to ease cooking and to provide the product with the desired white color. The germ is also removed because it contains oil, which contributes to shortened shelf life. Thus, the refined product is mainly composed of endosperm. Yet, it is the germ which provides much of the protein, vitamins, and minerals, and the bran which serves as an excellent source of fiber. Enrichment of refined grains replaces only four of the many nutrients and none of the fiber lost during processing. Whole-grain products are obviously a more nutritious option.

In selecting whole grain products, it is important to read labels carefully. A darkly colored product is not necessarily whole grain. Often foods are colored to resemble whole grain products, yet are actually highly refined and lacking in fiber content. The label of a product which is truly whole grain will include the term "whole" and/or "100%."

After careful examination of the sample food labels listed below, check (✓) the whole grain product in each pair. Which product in each pair would tend to contain the greatest fiber content?

☐ Wonder Wheat Bread: enriched wheat flour, cracked wheat, yeast, sugar, molasses, salt.
☐ Whole Wheat Bread: 100% whole wheat flour, shortening, yeast, salt.

☐ Super Granola Cereal: rolled oats, almonds, honey, vegetable oil, sea salt.
☐ Oatmeal: 100% rolled oats.

☐ Healthy Snack Crax: wheat flour, enriched flour, vegetable oil, dextrose, salt.
☐ Whole Rye Thins: 100% whole rye, vegetable oil, salt, sesame.

☐ Super Spaghetti: semolina, soya flour, wheat gluten, whey protein concentrate, calcium caseinate.
☐ Whole Wheat Noodles: 100% whole wheat flour, wheat germ, seven sprouted whole grains, salt.

☐ Enriched Long Grain Rice: pre-cooked long grain rice enriched with niacin, iron, thiamin, riboflavin.
☐ Brown Rice: long grain parboiled brown rice.

☐ Wheat Flour: enriched wheat.
☐ Whole Wheat Flour: 100% whole wheat.

The second choice in each pair contains or is 100% whole grain, so is less refined and higher in fiber than each of the first choices.

STEP 3: LET'S LIST THEM

Listed in the chart on page 80 are a variety of whole grains and whole grain products. Check (✓) those items which you have never eaten, those you tend to avoid, and those products which you do include in your diet. Note that some vegetables are nutritionally comparable to grains, so are included in the Grain Group rather than in the Fruit and Vegetable Group.

STEP 4: AVOID THE "NATURAL" FAD

Many products which have been identified as beneficial to health are seized upon by health pro-

moters and quacks and promoted as miracle cures for a variety of ills. As soon as the public learned of the possible role of fiber in the prevention of digestive diseases, "high fiber" products began to appear in health food stores and supermarkets across the nation—at high prices, of course.

Small amounts of cellulose, a common type of dietary fiber, are added to a variety of foods for several practical reasons:

• to ice cream to prevent crystal formation
• to whipped cream as a stabilizing agent
• to low-calorie salad dressings to prevent ingredient separation
• to diet soft drinks as a thickener

Certain bread manufacturers also began to advertise "high fiber" products, which actually contained added cellulose processed from wood pulp. Wood pulp fiber does not function in the same manner as the dietary fiber found in whole grains, fruits, and vegetables, and is unable to absorb the great quantities of water necessary for enhancing digestive function. The long range side effects from consuming significant quantities of wood pulp fiber are as yet unknown.

It is preferable and less costly to obtain the fiber needed for optimal digestive health simply by eating whole grains, and by including a variety of fruits and vegetables in the diet as well.

Select the whole grain products from the list below which are naturally high in fiber; check (✓) only those products which have not been fortified with added fiber:

☐ Superstuff Cereal—rolled oats, brown sugar, coconut oil, coconut, powdered cellulose,* almonds, honey.
☐ Oatmeal—100% rolled oats.
☐ Groovy Grain Bread—"organically grown" stone ground wheat* flour, water, eggs, honey, powdered cellulose*, vegetable shortening, yeast, salt, calcium sulfate, potassium bromate, potassium iodate.
☐ Rye Bread—100% whole wheat flour, water, whole rye flour, whole wheat kernels, salt, molasses, vegetable oil, yeast.
☐ Hi-Fiber Bread—water, flour, powdered cellulose*, wheat gluten, brown sugar, yeast, salt, sugar, soy flour, calcium sulfate, potassium bromate.

---

*"the plant fiber—finely powdered food grade cellulose—is refined from a naturally abundant wood source, and this cellulose is similar to that found in fruits, vegetables, and other common foods."

Whole Grain Product	Never Eaten (✓)	Tend to Avoid (✓)	Do Eat (✓)
barley			
buckwheat			
bulgur (cracked wheat)			
cornmeal			
kasha (cracked buckwheat)			
millet			
brown rice			
rolled oats			
rye flour			
sourdough (whole rye flour)			
tabouleh (bulgur wheat salad)			
triticale (wheat and rye)			
whole wheat flour			
shredded wheat cereal			
instant whole wheat cereal			
instant wheat and barley cereal			
whole wheat crackers			
stoned wheat crackers			
whole wheat matzoth			
wheat pilaf			
wheat berries			
whole wheat bread			
whole wheat waffles			
whole wheat English muffin			
whole wheat bagel			
whole wheat pasta (lasagna, noodles, spaghetti)			
couscous (semolina)			
tortilla (flat corn patty)			
taco (crispy corn patty)			
cornbread			
corn pone (whole corn cereal)			
corn muffin			
oatmeal bread			
rye bread			
whole rye crackers			
cream of rye cereal			
pumpernickel bread			
pumpernickel bagel			
pumpernickel melba toast			
sprouted grain cereal			
sprouted grain bread			
whole grain melba toast			
cracked wheat crackers			
whole grain granola cereal			

Note the brief description for some of the less common grain products in the chart above. A variety of delicious and nutritious recipes using whole grains are included in Days Twenty-One and Twenty-Three.

Oatmeal and rye bread are whole-grain products, while Superstuff Cereal, Groovy Grain Bread, and Hi-Fiber Bread have been refined and then fortified with cellulose so that their so-called "high fiber" contents can be promoted. Consumer beware! The fiber you want to include in your diet is not the added wood pulp found in the costly fortified "health" products. Rather, it is the dietary fiber found naturally in whole grain products and in fruits and vegetables.

STEP 5: GRAINS IN YOUR DIET

Do you think that you include the recommended number of grain servings in your daily diet? Are your Grain Group choices whole grain products, high in vitamins, minerals and fiber? Use your Nutri-Plan diet diary to determine whether your diet included the proper number of recommended servings from the Grain Group on Day Eleven. In the chart on page 81, list all grains consumed on Day Eleven, and total the number of servings. Do not forget to include the starchy vegetables listed in Day Eleven. Then, using product labels and the chart given in Step 3, check (✓) those items eaten which are whole grain products. Compare the totals. Did you include a majority of whole grain choices? And did you tend to select true whole grain products in preference to the more sugary, fatty, and/or fiber-fortified counterparts?

Remember that the grain content of your diet, when chosen wisely, can contribute many essential nutrients and fiber.

STEP 6: DAY TWELVE PLAN

Continue to record everything you eat and drink in your Nutri-Plan diet diary. For Day Twelve, continue to be aware of your nutrient intake. Try to approximate your personal needs, and to select foods wisely from the basic food groups; watch out for an excessive dependence on foods from the Others Group.

Day Eleven

Grain and Amount	Whole Grain (✔)

Total Grain Servings: _____
Total Whole Grain Servings: _____
No. Recommended Servings: <u>4 or more</u>

On Day Twelve, eat a whole grain product that you have never eaten before. You may want to choose a grain product from the chart in Step 3; do not be afraid to try out an unusual recipe (several recipes using whole grain products are given on Days Twenty-One and Twenty-Three). Then complete the grain questionnaire given below. Remember that grains, especially whole grains, can donate nutrients and fiber to your diet. And eating grains can be a healthfully delicious experience as well!

Grain Questionnaire

1) What new whole-grain product did you include in your diet on Day Twelve? _____

2) If possible, list product ingredients given on label: _____
_____

3) How was the product included in your diet (eg, as a plain bowl of cereal, cooked in a casserole, baked in a bread, etc)? _____

4) Did you like this new food? _____ Why or why not? _____
_____

5) Please add any additional comments you may want to make: _____
_____

DAY THIRTEEN

MILK AND CHEESE GROUP

STEP 1: COMPARING CHOICES

The typical American diet of today tends not to include enough milk or milk products and, although it was not mentioned in the *Dietary Goals, Dietary Guidelines,* or *Healthy People,* many of us do need to increase our intake of these foods. The basic food groups can guide us in the selection of:

- Two or more daily servings for adults.
- Three or more daily servings for children.
- Four or more daily servings for teens.

However, many people avoid milk and foods made with milk once reaching adulthood, succumbing instead to tempting selections from the Others Group. Milk is our best food source of the essential mineral calcium. The body requires calcium all throughout the lifespan, yet adults (especially females) tend to consider milk drinking as something which is eventually outgrown. And unfortunately, our bodies suffer from the inevitable damages.

In the list below, circle the food from each pair that you would be most likely to choose for a typical snack or as part of an average meal. The correct or wisest answer may seem obvious in some instances, but try to make your selections as honestly as possible—the wisest answers are usually not the most popular!

- bagel with part-skim mozzarella cheese or bagel with cream cheese
- coffee with skim milk or coffee with cream
- hamburger and skim milk or hamburger and cola
- pretzels and skim milk or pretzels and beer
- crackers and cottage cheese or chips and dip
- skim milk before dinner or martinis before dinner
- skim milk with dinner or wine with dinner
- skim milk and pie or coffee and pie
- berries with skim milk or berries with whipped cream

- vanilla yogurt or chocolate ice cream

Now compare the nutritional and caloric values for each of the selections in the pairs listed above. Perhaps the results will influence your food choices. It is simply a matter of nutritional priorities.

Food and Amount	Calories	Calcium (in milligrams)
mozzarella cheese, part-skim, 1 oz	80	207
cream cheese, 1 oz	106	18
skim milk, 2 oz	22	74
cream (light), 2 tbsp	64	30
skim milk, 8 oz	88	296
cola, 8 oz	96	0
skim milk, 8 oz	88	296
beer, 8 oz	101	12
cottage cheese, low-fat, ½ cup	82	70
dip, onion, 2 oz	116	56
skim milk, 8 oz	88	296
martinis, 4 oz (2)	224	0
skim milk, 8 oz	88	296
wine, red, 8 oz	328	16
skim milk, 8 oz	88	296
coffee with 2 tbsp cream (light)	64	30
skim milk, ½ cup	44	148
whipped cream, ½ cup	76	t
low-fat yogurt, vanilla, 1 cup	200	294
ice cream, chocolate, 1 cup	352	115

Caloric contents of the skim milk selections would double if whole milk was substituted. (Remember that fat provides more than twice as many calories per gram or per ounce as either carbohydrate or protein.) Milk is mainly composed of carbohydrate, plus a considerable amount of protein. And when the fat content is removed, the caloric value is reduced by half; since the fat-soluble vitamins are affected, select skim milk products which are fortified with vitamins A and D.

Although the addition of sugar does not increase the caloric content as much as the addition of fat, the sugar calories are not accompanied by vitamins and minerals. Thus, sweetened milk products have extra calories, but lack nutrient enhancement.

Look below in order to compare skim milk with the higher fat product whole milk, and also with the higher fat (plus added sugar) product ice cream. When the choice is yours, why not opt for the nutrient-rich, low-calorie selections?

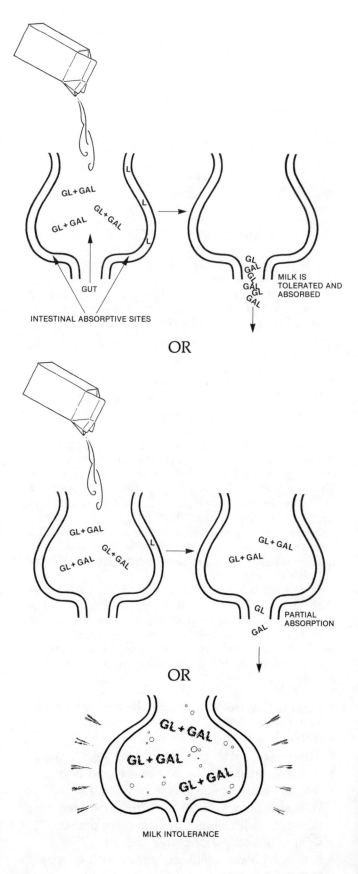

	Skim Milk (1 cup)	Whole Milk (1 cup)	Ice Cream (1 cup)
Calories	88	159	350
Protein	8.8 grams	8.5 grams	4.0 grams
Carbohydrate	12.5 grams	12.0 grams	14.7 grams
Fat	.2 grams	8.5 grams	24.0 grams
Cholesterol	4 mg	33 mg	88 mg
Vitamin A	500 IU	310 IU	900 IU
Riboflavin (B_2)	.37 mg	.40 mg	.28 mg
Calcium	296 mg	288 mg	115 mg

STEP 2: MILK INTOLERANCES

Some people do not drink milk for reasons other than ignorance about the nutritional contributions and/or confusion over bodily requirements. In fact, many people are actually unable to tolerate milk. And although milk intolerance has been recognized for centuries, the most common cause has only recently been identified.

Remember that lactose or milk sugar is a disaccharide (double sugar) composed of the simple sugars glucose and galactose. The disaccharide must be split into these simple sugar components in order to be absorbed from the gut. The enzyme (chemical assistant) required for this splitting process is called lactase. If the body contains an insufficient supply of lactase, any lactose presented to the gut is not properly broken down and absorbed. Instead, the lactose remains in the digestive tract, drawing in fluids and bacteria, and resulting in the intestinal discomforts of distention, "gas," cramps, and diarrhea. No wonder some people tend to avoid milk!

The following diagrams provide a simplified illustration of milk tolerance as compared to milk intolerance:

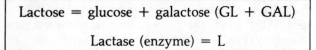

Lactose = glucose + galactose (GL + GAL)

Lactase (enzyme) = L

STEP 3: WHO CAN'T AND HOW MUCH?

Disorders other than lactase deficiency can also cause milk intolerance, such as a cows' milk allergy or a casein (milk protein) allergy. Lactase deficiency, however, is the most common reason for milk intolerance, and is apparently an inherited disorder. The following chart depicts the general distribution of this widespread nuisance:

Age Group	Race	Percent of Population Afflicted
11 months to 11 years	US Caucasian	10
	US Black	35
Adult	US Black	70
	Greek Cypriots	60 to 80
	Arab	60 to 80
	Ashkenazic Jew	60 to 80
	Japanese	over 90
	Thai	over 90
	Bantu	over 90
	Formosan	over 90
	Filipino	over 90
	Scandinavian	1 to 2

Over 70% of the world's population develops lactase deficiency by adulthood. Except for North and West European Caucasians, their descendants living in the US, and several other population groups, most of the world's adults are unable to tolerate milk.

Luckily, the lactose intolerant need not eliminate milk entirely, nor must they avoid all foods from the Milk and Cheese Group. Studies indicate that most people who have a lactase deficiency are able to tolerate moderate amounts of milk. In fact, the lactase deficient adult can usually drink one cup of milk per day without significant side effects, while most children appear to tolerate even larger amounts. Milk is best tolerated if it is:

• taken in small amounts (one cup or less)
• distributed throughout the day
• consumed with meals

Alternative selections from the Milk and Cheese Group contain less lactose than milk and are usually well tolerated. Individuals vary in their abilities to tolerate milk and milk products. Thus, it is important to gradually test personal tolerances for:

• yogurt
• cottage cheese
• cheese (aged cheddar is often well tolerated)

• milk (in small amounts) and foods made with milk

Lactose-free milk is also now available in many supermarkets.

STEP 4: LET'S LIST THEM

Listed in the chart on page 86 are a variety of milk products. Check (✓) those items which you have never consumed, those you tend to avoid, and those products which you do include in your diet.

Keep in mind the fact that certain items, indicated by an asterisk (*), have considerable fat and calorie content (unless made with skim milk); you may want to use a calorie chart (see Appendix C) to determine these values before including these particular (*) products in your diet. Also remember that cottage cheese and ice cream are lower in calcium contents than milk and hard cheeses.

A variety of nutritious and delicious recipes using milk products are included in Day Twenty-One and Day Twenty-Three. If you have a lactase deficiency, try experimenting with mealtime intakes of small amounts of milk and milk products. And remember, your body never outgrows the need for calcium-rich milk!

STEP 5: BETTER BY BREAST?

Milk intake is important all throughout the lifespan. However, milk is probably most essential during infancy when serving as the major, if not sole source of nutrients and calories. Indicate by check (✓) whether you think each of the following statements is true or false.

Compared to the bottle-fed infant, the breast-fed infant receives:

True False

☐ ☐ 1) better overall nutrition.
☐ ☐ 2) a larger dietary intake of cholesterol.
☐ ☐ 3) better quality protein.
☐ ☐ 4) iron in a form which is more readily absorbed.
☐ ☐ 5) extra anti-infection and anti-allergy benefits.
☐ ☐ 6) the psychological benefits of strong mother/infant interaction.
☐ ☐ 7) immunity against any drugs taken by the mother.

Except for the last one (7), all of the above statements are True, and provide the basis upon which professionals have established the general recommendation that infants be breast-fed whenever possible:

- Breast milk tends to be better absorbed and has a more desirable nutritional composition than formulas.
- The higher cholesterol content of breast milk may lead to improved cholesterol metabolism and decreased cholesterol build-up later in life.
- Protein level and quality of breast milk may be advantageous for infant growth and development.
- Heat-treated iron formulas and breast milk provide a more absorbable form of iron than cows' milk.
- Respiratory and other infections are less common in the breast-fed, while early exposure to cows' milk may be related to the development of allergies later in life.
- Breast-fed infants enjoy the strong mother/infant interaction which is of major importance in psychological and behavioral development.
- Most drugs taken by the lactating mother—including alcohol and caffeine—do appear in breast milk, making physician approval for any medication mandatory for the nursing mother.

The practice of breastfeeding has recently resurged in popularity, although some women are physically incapable and the working woman may find it inconvenient. However, behavioral and nutritional studies currently indicate that breastfeeding should be the method of choice, providing mental and physical health benefits to all infants, plus possible life-saving advantages for those in underdeveloped areas where economics and sanitation must be considered as well.

Milk Product	Never Eaten (✔)	Tend to Avoid (✔)	Do Eat (✔)
yogurt, plain, low-fat			
yogurt, flavored*			
yogurt, whole milk*			
cottage cheese, dry or low-fat			
cottage cheese, creamed*			
lactose-free milk			
ice milk*			
ice cream*			
milkshake*			
blenderized shake (skim milk, fruit, ice)			
non-fat dried milk powder			
puddings*			
custard*			
goats' milk			
chocolate milk*			
hot chocolate*			
evaporated milk, skim			
evaporated milk, whole*			
canned milk (evaporated, unsweetened)			
malted milk*			
macaroni and cheese*			
eggnog*			
cheese souffle*			
quiche (with cheese)*			
cheese soup*			
creamed soups (with milk)*			
chowders (with milk)*			
tapioca cream pudding*			
pizza*			
Welsh rarebit*			
cheese sauce*			
cheese-baked potatoes*			
kefir (yogurt drink)			

STEP 6: MILK AND CHEESE IN YOUR DIET

Do you think that you include the recommended number of milk product servings in your daily diet? Are your Milk and Cheese Group choices low in calories, but high in calcium and other nutrients? Use your Nutri-Plan diet diary to determine whether your diet included the proper number of recommended servings from the Milk and Cheese Group on Day Twelve. In the chart below, list all milk products consumed on Day Twelve, and total the number of servings. Were most of these prod-

ucts low in calories and fat? You may want to refer to the chart in Step 4 and to a nutrient values chart (see Appendix C) to help you determine this. Compare the totals. Also, did you tend to choose Milk and Cheese Group selections in preference to Others Group items?

When selected from wisely, the Milk and Cheese Group can provide sufficient calcium, plus other essential nutrients, without contributing excessive calories and fat. It is up to you to select the low-fat, nutritious Milk and Cheese Group products now available in a variety of delicious forms.

Day Twelve

Milk Product and Amount	High Calorie/Fat (✔)

Total Milk Product Servings: _____
Total High Calorie/Fat Servings: _____
No. Recommended Servings: _2 or more_ (adult) _3 or more_ (child) _4 or more_ (teen)

STEP 7: DAY THIRTEEN PLAN

Continue to record everything you eat and drink in your Nutri-Plan diet diary. For Day Thirteen, continue to be aware of your nutrient intake. Try to approximate your personal needs, and to select foods wisely from the basic food groups; watch out for an excessive dependence on foods from the Others Group.

On Day Thirteen, try a milk product that you have never consumed before. You may want to choose an item from the list in Step 4; do not be afraid to test out an unusual recipe (many recipes including milk products are given on Day Twenty-One and Day Twenty-Three). Try to choose a low-calorie, low-fat milk product in preference to the caloric, fat-rich items. Then complete the milk product questionnaire given below. Note: If you have a lactose deficiency, check with your physician before attempting to add even small amounts of milk products to your diet.

Remember, low-fat milk products are an especially wise way to calcium-enrich your diet.

Milk Product Questionnaire

1) What new milk product did you include in your diet on Day Thirteen? _____
_____

2) Using the food label and/or a nutrient values chart (see Appendix C), determine the number of calories and grams of fat in one serving of your new milk product: _____
How does this compare with one serving of skim milk? _____

3) How was the product included in your diet (eg, plain, blenderized drink, mixed into salad or casserole, baked in bread, etc)? _____
_____

4) Did you like this new food? _____ Why or why not? _____
_____

5) Please add any additional comments you may want to make: _____
_____

DAY FOURTEEN

MEAT AND ALTERNATES GROUP

STEP 1: COMPARING CHOICES

One of the dietary changes suggested by the *Dietary Goals, Dietary Guidelines,* and *Healthy People* is a decreased consumption of foods high in saturated fat and cholesterol, which requires wise food selection, particularly from the Meat and Alternates Group. The basic food groups can guide us in the selection of two or more daily servings. Unfortunately, most Americans tend to consume at least twice this amount, and place a hearty emphasis on red meat choices. By recalling the information given on Day Four, you know that meat can provide significant amounts of both saturated fat and cholesterol, which have been implicated in elevated blood lipid levels and associated health detriments.

In the list below, circle the food from each pair that you would be most likely to choose for a typical snack or as part of an average meal. The correct or wisest answer may seem obvious in some instances, but try to make your selections as honestly as possible—the wisest answers are usually not the most popular!

- broiled chicken or Porterhouse steak
- yogurt and fruit or cheeseburger and French fries
- oatmeal with milk or bacon and eggs
- baked halibut or lamb chops
- tuna fish sandwich or ham and cheese sandwich
- shredded wheat cereal or cheese omelet
- lentil casserole or beef stroganoff
- eggplant submarine sandwich or roast beef submarine sandwich
- peanut butter on whole wheat bread or hot dog on roll
- tossed salad with chickpeas and peanuts or with bacon bits

Now compare the caloric and fat values for each of the selections in the pairs listed above with the chart on page 90. Perhaps the results will influence your food choices. It is simply a matter of nutritional priorities.

Remember that fat provides more than twice as many calories per gram or per ounce as either carbohydrate or protein. Thus, meat selections often contain such a high percentage of fat that they are actually poor protein foods: the amount of protein provided is outweighed by the excessive fat/caloric content.

When the choice is yours, why not opt for the low-calorie, low-fat meats and alternates?

STEP 2: TRIM THEM DOWN

Some of the visible fat can be trimmed from meat products and their alternates in order to lower the total fat (and caloric) contents. Look at the chart on page 90 which compares some typical meat cuts (cooked) and alternate products to their defatted counterparts. Note the difference in total calories and fat calories once each item is trimmed of visible fat.

To decrease the fat and calorie contributions of your meat and alternates group selections, try incorporating some of the following suggestions into your present food purchasing and preparation methods:

- Choose meats with the least amounts of visible white fat.
- Ask that all meat be trimmed before being ground—"hamburger" may include added beef fat, "ground beef" has no added fat; note percentage of fat on labels.
- Before cooking, trim all meats of visible white fat.
- Remove skin from poultry prior to cooking; try ground turkey as a meat extender.
- Bake, boil, broil, or roast on wire rack (to allow excess fat to drain)—never fry; avoid the addition of fat during preparation.
- Obviously, raw meat weighs more than trimmed, boned, cooked meats; allow for the

following average serving amounts when pur-
chasing raw meat—
  Boneless—¼ to ⅓ pound per serving.
  Bone-in—⅓ to ½ pound per serving.
  Bony (ribs)—¾ to 1 pound per serving.

Again, when the choice is yours, why not make your selections low-fat and calorie-smart? Be heart-wise and heart-healthy!

Food and Amount	Calories	Fat (in grams)
chicken, broiled (without skin)	206	5.5
Porterhouse steak, 4 oz	400	37.2
yogurt, low-fat, 1 cup	123	4.2
hamburg, 3 oz + American cheese, 1 oz	235 + 105 = 340	16.6 + 8.8 = 25.4
oatmeal, 1 cup + milk, skim, ½ cup	312 + 44 = 356	5.9 + .1 = 6.0
bacon, 2 slices + eggs, fried, 2	172 + 198 = 370	15.6 + 15.8 = 31.4
halibut, baked, 4 oz	192	8.0
lamb chops, 3.1 oz	362	31.7
tuna fish salad, commercial, ½ cup	175	10.8
ham, 2 oz + Swiss cheese, 1 oz	112 + 105 = 217	9.6 + 7.9 = 17.5
shredded wheat, 1 biscuit + milk, skim, ½ cup	89 + 44 = 133	.5 + .1 = .6
omelet (2 eggs) + cheese, cheddar, 1½ oz	222 + 170 = 392	16.6 + 13.6 = 30.2
lentils, ½ cup + whole wheat noodles, ½ cup	106 + 98 = 204	t + t = t
beef, chuck, 1 cup + noodles, ½ cup + gravy, 1 tbsp	458 + 100 + 28 = 586	33.5 + 1.2 + 1.2 = 35.9
eggplant, steamed, 1 cup + part-skim mozzarella cheese, 1 oz	38 + 80 = 118	.4 + 5 = 5.4
roast beef, lean with fat, 3 oz	374	33.5
peanut butter, 1 tbsp + whole wheat bread, 1 slice	94 + 61 = 155	8.1 + .8 = 8.9
frankfurter, 1 sm	139	12.4
chickpeas, 1 tbsp + peanuts, 1 tbsp	45 + 52 = 97	.6 + 4.4 = 5.0
bacon bits, 1 oz	165	13.5

Meat or Alternate	Amount	Total Calories	Fat Calories
Beans, dried, with pork and sauce	⅔ cup	210	40
Beans, dried (canned)	⅔ cup	155	6
Beef, ground, medium (21% fat)	3 oz	240	150
Beef, ground, lean (10% fat)	3 oz	190	90
Beef, rib roast, untrimmed	6 oz	430	220
Beef, rib roast, trimmed	6 oz	300	80
Cheese, cottage, creamed (4.2% milk fat)	½ cup	110	80
Cheese, cottage, uncreamed	½ cup	60	2
Chicken, with skin	4 oz	255	70
Chicken, without skin	4 oz	200	64
Egg, fried	1 large	100	70
Egg, poached or boiled	1 large	80	50
Fish, fried (breaded, frozen)	4 oz	300	180
Fish, broiled	4 oz	190	20
Lamb, loin chops, untrimmed	5.3 oz	340	250
Lamb, loin chops, trimmed	5.3 oz	120	40
Pork, spareribs, untrimmed	6.3 oz	790	630
Pork, loin chops, untrimmed	5 oz	610	440
Pork, loin chops, trimmed	5 oz	300	150
Scallops, fried (breaded, frozen)	4 oz	210	80
Scallops, broiled	4 oz	120	15
Shrimp, fried (breaded)	3 oz	190	80
Shrimp, uncooked	3 oz	90	10
Tuna fish salad (with mayonnaise)	½ cup	180	100
Tuna, canned in oil	3 oz	150	60
Tuna, water-packed	3 oz	120	8

STEP 3: SO WHAT ARE THE ALTERNATIVES?

Every living cell contains protein—skin, muscle, blood, hair, heart, brain, nerves, etc. Protein is essential to growth, health, and life itself. A diet high in protein usually contains abundant amounts of animal foods (meat, poultry, fish, eggs, milk, cheese).

Animal foods provide high quality protein, but some believe that such products are agriculturally extravagant, since turning plants into animal foods uses a significant amount of land, which can be quite costly. In fact, for almost as long as man has been eating meat, someone has opposed the practice; vegetarianism can be traced as far back as the early biblical days.

There is little reason for you to avoid all animal foods. Moderate quantities can provide high quality protein, plus a variety of essential vitamins and minerals. Without animal foods, a diet is likely to be lacking in vitamin B_{12} and low in iron content. Due to an increased awareness concerning the saturated fat and cholesterol contents of meats, different degrees of vegetarianism are now practiced by the health conscious. Coupled with today's high costs for meats and most other animal products, the elimination or decreased intake of animal foods has become increasingly appealing.

From the following, select the term which best describes your present eating habits. Do you want to increase or decrease your total meat consumption? Do you think that such a dietary change could be of any benefit to your present or future health?

In addition to plant foods (fruits, vegetables, grains, legumes, nuts, and seeds), the:

- Non-vegetarian consumes meat and other animal products on a regular basis.

- Semi-vegetarian consumes poultry, fish, eggs, and milk products, but avoids red meats.
- Lacto-ovo vegetarian consumes eggs and dairy products (eg, Seventh Day Adventists).
- Lacto-vegetarian consumes dairy products (eg, Trappist monks).
- Vegan avoids all animal products.

Most vegetarians are able to obtain all of the essential nutrients, if they are appropriately educated on the subject and particularly careful in food selection. Vegetarianism-related nutritional problems have been detected, however, especially amongst:

- infants
- children
- pregnant women
- restrictive vegans or fad-followers (eg, macrobiotics, fruitarians)

In those instances where nutrient needs are not being met through dietary means, nutritional supplementation may be prescribed by the physician. Remember that variety in food selection is essential for a nutritious, well-balanced diet.

STEP 4: PROS and CONS FOR NON-MEAT EATING

The chart below lists some of the positive and negative factors associated with meatless diets. In order to determine whether you may want to alter the Meat and Alternates Group portion of your present diet, check (✔) those possible pros which you consider to be personally important. Then check (✔) the possible cons which are also of considerable importance to you. Total your pros; then

Possible Pros (✔) (for adoption of a well-balanced, non-meat diet)		Possible Cons (✔) (for adoption of a well-balanced, non-meat diet)	
I want to lower my blood cholesterol level.	☐	I may require supplementation (since I am an infant/child/ pregnant woman).	☐
I want to lower my blood pressure.	☐	I may develop nutritional deficiencies (since I am/will become a restrictive vegetarian).	☐
I want to lower my overall risks for developing heart disease.	☐	I may develop caloric deficiencies (since I am an infant/ child/pregnant woman/underweight person/problem eater).	☐
I want to lower my risks for developing other diseases of higher incidence in meat eating countries (eg, cancer of the breast and colon).	☐	I may encounter burdensome social difficulties (at restaurants, dinner parties, family meals, etc).	☐
I want to lose weight.	☐	I may encounter difficulties with increasing meal frequency (less dietary fat can cause more frequent hunger pangs).	☐
I want to lessen the incidence of constipation.	☐	I may dislike the need for frequenting the bathroom more often (due to increased dietary fiber).	☐
I want to decrease my food bills.	☐	I may dislike the need for special care in food selection and preparation.	☐
Total Pros: _____		Total Cons: _____	

total your cons and compare the results. Are changes in your selections from the Meat and Alternates Group advisable at this time? Are you going to make these changes?

STEP 5: TO BE OR NOT TO BE...

☑ YES If you decide to try out the vegetarian way of life, be sure to avoid food faddism, and include a wide variety of foods in your diet. You need not purchase expensive self-prescribed supplements, nor adhere to a severely restrictive diet plan. A well-balanced diet which includes a variety of nutritious food choices can easily fit into the semi-vegetarian or the lacto-ovo vegetarian lifestyle. As you begin to decrease your consumption of meat, keep in mind the following suggestions:

- Be sure to obtain a sufficient amount of vitamin B_{12} through intake of some animals foods, fortified soy/special yeast products, or physician-prescribed supplements.
- Include sufficient dietary iron, especially during infancy, childhood, and pregnancy; note that the phytates present in whole grain products can inhibit iron absorption.
- Meet all nutrient needs by selecting nutritious foods in preference to the high-calorie, sugary/fatty choices.
- Only take nutritional supplements if prescribed by a physician; infants, children, and pregnant women are particularly susceptible to nutrient deficiencies and may require closer medical supervision.

Now, use the chart below to assist you in planning meals and snacks which contain high quality protein and minimal fat. Remember that plant foods do not provide high quality protein, but certain combinations of proteins—from different plants, or from plant foods with animal foods—may complement one another so as to contribute protein of good quality (see Day Two for a review, if necessary).

Note: You may want to use the plant food definitions given below for further assistance.

Plant Food Definitions:
Grains include barley, buckwheat, bulgur, corn, millet, oats, rice, rye, wheat and their products.
Legumes include black beans, broad beans, chickpeas, cowpeas, dried peas, kidney beans, lentils, lima beans, mung beans, navy beans, pea beans, soybeans, tofu, white beans.
Nuts include black walnuts, Brazil nuts, cashews, peanuts, and pistachios.
Seeds include pumpkin, sesame, squash, and sunflower seeds.

☑ NO If you decide not to opt for a vegetarian lifestyle, you may want to consider the following suggestions:

- Diet plays an important role in determining your state of health and well-being.
- Dietary fat and cholesterol may have an effect on your health.
- Meats and other animal products contain varying amounts of fat and cholesterol.
- Be moderate in your consumption of animal foods, particularly those high in fat and/or cholesterol.

The next two steps identify those foods which can contribute significant amounts of fat and/or cholesterol to the diet. As always, the choice is yours—why not make your food selections wise ones?

STEP 6: LET'S LIST THEM

Without any fat at all, meat would taste very different: it would be noticeably tougher, drier, and less appetizing. Since fat provides satiety value, a fat-free meat cut would be swiftly digested and unsatisfying to our stomachs and our palates.
There are no meat cuts which contain absolutely no fat. Today's cuts, however, tend to have more

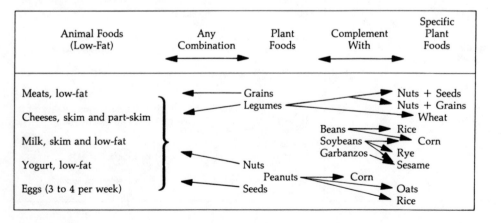

lean in proportion to fat and bone. This is because meat retailers and packers now trim off more fat, while today's herders raise cattle, hogs, and sheep in such a way that less fat is produced; fat content is relative to the age of the animal, and to the type and amount of animal feed.

Cuts from an animal's hindquarters tend to have less fat than those from the forequarters. These leaner cuts of meat, when properly prepared, can be appetizing, tender, and more nutritious than the fattier cuts. Ounce for ounce, lean meats have more protein, vitamins, and minerals—yet less caloric and fat contents than fattier meats.

In the chart below, a variety of meats have been divided into three different categories on the basis of fat content. It may be healthier and more economical to select from the low-fat category; note that the medium-fat choices are popular, and make wiser selections than the high-fat items. Note that those products indicated by an asterisk (*) are especially high in cholesterol.

Obviously, the wisest choices are from the low-fat category. In selecting meat as part of your two or more daily servings from the Meat and Alternates Group, note the following:

- Fat category—is it a low-fat, medium-fat, or high-fat choice?
- Visible fat—did you trim off all visible white fat and/or skin?
- Preparation—did you bake, boil, broil, or roast on a rack without any added fats?
- Cholesterol—is it a high-cholesterol choice (*)?

STEP 7: HIGH-CHOLESTEROL FOODS

Most people are aware that meat contains an appreciable amount of cholesterol. All animal foods, in fact, contain cholesterol. Therefore, even vegetarians (except vegans) are susceptible to excessive cholesterol intakes. If the blood becomes overloaded with cholesterol and certain other lipids, plaques begin to form along the blood vessel walls. The plaques clog and narrow blood vessels, forcing the heart to work harder than normal in order to pump the blood through. If a main blood vessel leading to the heart becomes entirely blocked off, a heart attack results. If a vessel leading to the brain is blocked, a stroke occurs. Blockage of blood vessels in the legs causes claudication with the resultant leg pain and numbness.

Low-Fat Meats	Medium-Fat Meats	High-Fat Meats

Beef
   Steak: Flank, bottom round,
       top round
   Roast: Tip
   Pot Roast: Heel of round
   Ground: Extra lean
	Beef
	   Steak: Porterhouse, rib,
	       sirloin, T-bone,
	       tenderloin
	   Pot Roast: Arm, blade, boneless neck
	       (rolled), standing rump
	   Ground beef
	   Stew meat: Round
		Beef
		   Steak: Top loin
		   Roast: Rib
		   Brisket
		   Short ribs
		   Stew meat: Chuck

Veal
   Chop: Loin, rib
   Steak: Arm, blade, cutlet, sirloin
   Roast: Rump, sirloin
		Veal
		   Stew meat: Breast

Pork
   Leg (fresh ham)
	Pork
	   Chop: Loin center cut
	   Steak: Blade
	   Roast: Arm picnic shoulder, ham-rump
	       and shank, sirloin, tenderloin
	   Canadian bacon
		Pork
		   Roast: Blade, butt, loin
		       and shoulder,
		       smoked arm picnic
		   Spareribs

Lamb
   Leg roast
	Lamb
	   Chop: Arm, loin
		Lamb
		   Chop: Blade, rib
		   Riblets

Cured
   Dried beef
		Cured
		   Bacon, bologna, corned beef, frankfurter,
		       headcheese, liver sausage, salami, sausage

Variety*
   Brain, Heart, Kidney, Liver, Sweetbreads
		Variety
		   Tongue

Poultry
   Chicken (without skin)
   Turkey (without skin)
		Poultry
		   Capon, duck, goose

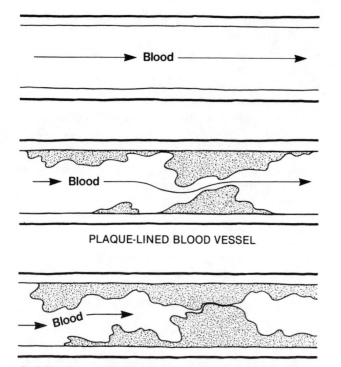

PLAQUE-LINED BLOOD VESSEL

BLOCKAGE = HEART ATTACK, STROKE, CLAUDICATION

Diet may have a direct effect on the blood levels of cholesterol and certain other lipids. In combination with other risk factors, the composition of your diet may play an essential role in the prevention or development of the following disorders:

- atherosclerosis
- hyperlipidemia
- coronary artery disease
- heart attack
- stroke
- claudication
- circulatory problems

The degree to which diet actually contributes to these disorders is currently under investigation and is often the subject of heated debates. However, it is generally accepted that certain dietary components tend to lead to specific observable effects:

- high level of saturated fat in the diet → ↑ blood levels of fats and cholesterol
- high level of cholesterol in the diet → ↑ blood levels of fats and cholesterol
- ↓ dietary intake of fats and cholesterol → ↓ blood levels of fats and cholesterol

Note: The presence of large amounts of HDL, a certain type of blood cholesterol factor, may prove to be beneficial, and may play a protective role against cholesterol build-up. Research indicates that the blood levels of HDLs (high density lipoproteins) may be elevated through increased physical activity, loss of excess body weight, and moderate alcohol intake—if nothing else, at least this prescription can make you look and feel better!

On Day Four, you identified the dietary sources of saturated fat. You have also become aware that the *Dietary Goals*, *Dietary Guidelines*, and *Healthy People* suggest a decreased intake of foods high in fat, especially saturated fat. Careful selection of foods from the Milk and Cheese Group and from the Meat and Alternates Group, in conjunction with a limited intake of the Others Group foods, can contribute to the desired moderation in the consumption of saturated fat.

Dietary cholesterol can also be minimized, simply through moderation in the consumption of high-cholesterol foods. The chart below may assist you in the identification of those foods which contain considerable amounts of cholesterol.

High-Cholesterol Foods			
Animal fats	Cold cuts	Hamburger	Quail
Bacon	Cream	Heart*	Rabbit
Beans and franks, canned	Cream cheese	Ice cream	Roe
Beef, fatty cuts	Cream puff	Kidney*	Salt pork
Beef and vegetable stew	Cream, sour	Lamb, fatty cuts	Sauce, cheese
Beef, corned	Cream, whipped	Lard	Sausage
Beef pot pie	Custard	Liver*	Shrimp*
Boston cream pie	Duck	Luncheon meats	Soups, creamed
Brains*	Eggs*	Milk, condensed	Spareribs
Butter	Eggnog	Milk, evaporated	Sweetbreads*
Caviar	Frankfurters	Milk, whole	Tongue
Cheese, unless part-skim or skim	Giblets	Pate de foie gras*	Tripe
Chicken pot pie	Goose, domestic	Pigs' feet	Veal, fatty cuts
Chili con carne	Gravies	Pork, fatty cuts	Yogurt, from whole milk

*Especially high

STEP 8: CHOLESTEROL IN YOUR DIET

Do you think that you include too much cholesterol in your daily diet? How much cholesterol did you consume each day in the past? The *Dietary Goals* suggest a daily intake of approximately 300 milligrams. Use your Nutri-Plan diet diary and a nutrient values chart (see Appendix C) in order to determine just how many milligrams of cholesterol were provided by your diet on Day One. In the chart below, list all foods and beverages consumed on Day One and the amounts. Use the chart in Step 7 to check (✓) those items eaten which are high in cholesterol; determine the approximate number of milligrams of cholesterol provided by each of these high-cholesterol (✓) items. Total the approximate number of milligrams of cholesterol included in your diet on Day One. Did you include more or less than the number of milligrams suggested for daily intake? Do you think that you have improved your diet from the standpoint of cholesterol intake since Day One?

Day One

Food and Amount	High Cholesterol (✓)	Amount of Cholesterol (in milligrams)

Total Cholesterol Intake:_____mg
Suggested Daily Cholesterol Intake:___300___mg

Note: Your results are merely an estimate to be used for illustrative purposes only, since the available data on the cholesterol contents of most foods is still incomplete, and actual cholesterol absorption varies among individuals.

STEP 9: MEAT AND ALTERNATES IN YOUR DIET

Do you think that you include the recommended number of meat and alternates servings in your daily diet? Are your choices low in saturated fat and cholesterol? Use your Nutri-Plan diet diary in order to determine whether your diet included the proper number of recommended servings from the Meat and Alternates Group on Day Thirteen, and if your choices were low in fat and cholesterol.

In the chart below, list all meat and alternates consumed on Day Thirteen and the amounts. Using the charts in Steps 6 and 7, and the chart on sources of saturated fat in Day Four, check (✓) the high-fat and the high-cholesterol items. Total each column and compare the results. Did you tend to choose the low-fat, cholesterol-free products in preference to the high-fat, cholesterol-rich animal foods? The Meat and Alternates Group can provide both the vegetarian and the meat eater with many needed nutrients, while the fat and cholesterol contributions can be minimized by:

- careful selection.
- proper preparation.
- moderation in consumption.

Day Thirteen

Meat and Alternates and Amounts	High Fat (✓)	High Colesterol (✓)

Total Meat and Alternate Servings:_____
No. Recommended Servings:___2____

Total High-Fat:_____
Total High-Cholesterol:_____

STEP 10: DAY FOURTEEN PLAN

Continue to record everything that you eat and drink in your Nutri-Plan diet diary. For Day Fourteen, continue to be aware of your nutrient intake. Select foods wisely from the basic food groups, and avoid overemphasis on items from the Others Group.

At the end of Day Fourteen, complete another chart to total your cholesterol intake for Day Fourteen using the methods you utilized in Step 8. Compare your total cholesterol intake with the daily intake amount suggested by the *Dietary Goals* (300 mg); then compare to your total cholesterol intake for Day One (from Step 8). Have you improved since Day One? Let's hope that by now you are cholesterol wise!

The Meat and Alternates Group offers a wide variety of nutritious food choices, some more moderate in fat, calorie, and cholesterol contents than others. Vegetarianism can prove to be a healthy choice, but only with careful food selection in order to meet all nutrient needs. Your food choices from the Meat and Alternates Group, like your decisions regarding meat eating versus vegetarianism, can have quite an influence over your overall health and well-being, now and in the future. The choice is yours, so have a heart—a healthy heart!

DAY FIFTEEN

OTHERS GROUP

STEP 1: COMPARING CHOICES

The *Dietary Goals, Dietary Guidelines,* and *Healthy People* suggested a decrease in the consumption of fat, sugar, and salt and the intake of calories in amounts necessary for maintenance of desirable weight. The *Dietary Guidelines* and *Healthy People* also recommend moderation in alcohol intake. Yet, in America today, the intake of fat, sugar, salt, calories, and alcohol continues to be excessive, and the consequences are visible. The Others Group includes foods high in fat, sugar, salt, and/or alcohol; these products contain considerable calories with little, if any, accompanying nutrients. And unfortunately, our diets tend to include an abundance of selections from the Others Group.

In the list below, circle the food from each pair that you would be most likely to choose for a typical snack or as part of an average meal. The correct or wisest answer may seem obvious in some instances, but try to make your selections as honestly as possible—the wisest answers are usually not the most popular!

- whole wheat bagel or glazed donut
- fresh cherries or cherry pie
- fruit salad or banana cream pie
- orange juice or cola
- mineral water or draught beer
- club soda or rosé wine
- tossed salad or potato chips
- coleslaw or French fried potatoes
- lettuce and tomato or pickle spears
- yogurt or onion dip

Now compare the caloric and nutrient values for each of the selections in the pairs listed above to the chart on page 100. Note which selections contain considerable amounts of fat, sugar, salt, and/or alcohol. Perhaps the results will influence your food choices. It is simply a matter of nutritional priorities.

Note that fried and fatty foods usually provide many calories and little nutrient value. (Remember that fat provides more than twice as many calories per gram or per ounce as either carbohydrate or protein.) Foods high in added sugar usually have an abundance of calories with little, if any, accompanying nutrients—and these foods taste so good that we tend to overeat them. Foods high in salt are often too low in nutrient value to offset the excessive sodium contents. Alcoholic beverages also offer more calories than nutrients; approaching fat in caloric value, alcohol provides seven calories per gram. And those who drink alcohol regularly and excessively may require more nutrients to maintain good health than those who do not imbibe.

Obviously, it is up to you to make wise food choices and to use extra care in selecting from the Others Group.

STEP 2: "OTHERS" DEFINED

What causes a food or beverage to be considered as an Others Group product? In general, those foods that are high in calories, yet low in nutrient value are the main components of this additional basic food group. These foods contain considerable amounts of one or more of the following:

Food and Amount	Calories	High In:
bagel, whole wheat	160	fiber, B-vitamins, iron, phosphorus, magnesium
donut, glazed	205	fat, sugar
cherries, 1 cup	60	fiber, vitamin A
cherry pie, ⅛ of pie	308	fat, sugar
fruit salad, fresh, 1 cup	86	fiber, vitamin C, potassium
banana cream pie, ⅛ of pie	252	fat, sugar
orange juice, fresh, 1 cup	112	vitamin C, potassium
cola, 12 oz can	144	sugar
mineral water, 12 oz	0	trace minerals, water
beer, 12 oz	156	alcohol
club soda, 12 oz	0	water
wine, rosé, 3½ oz	141	alcohol
tossed salad (lettuce, cucumber, tomato, sprouts)	35	fiber, vitamin A, folic acid, potassium
potato chips, 15	171	fat, salt
coleslaw (vinegar type), ½ cup	114	fiber, vitamin C, potassium
French fried potatoes, 15	321	fat, salt
lettuce and tomato, 2 to 3 slices	12	fiber, vitamin A, potassium
dill pickles, 4 spears	12	salt
yogurt, low-fat, ½ cup	57	B-vitamins, calcium
onion dip (sour cream base), ½ cup	140	fat, salt

- Fat
- Sugar
- Salt
- Alcohol

For each of the Others Group foods, the detriments outweigh any possible nutritional benefits. In fact, the Others Group contains many items which damage health rather than enhance it. Yet, each year the American diet includes more and more selections from the Others Group. These foods are not meant to compose our diet, but only to complement it! Let's take a look at the statistics:

- The average American diet in 1976 contained 31% more dietary fat than in 1910.
- The average American diet in 1976 contained 50% more refined sugar than in 1910.
- Most Americans today consume at least 5 times more salt (sodium) than needed.
- Alcohol abuse remains one of our major killers, as well as an important cause of nutritional deficiencies in our country today.

We could do ourselves a healthy favor by minimizing the intake of these high-calorie, low-nutrient foodstuffs. Unfortunately, this is far easier said than done. Food habits are difficult to change because they are often a very personal aspect of our lives.

On Day Eight, you listed ten of your favorite foods. In the chart on page 101, relist these ten items and indicate why your Others Group favorites are considered as such. A sample has been illustrated for you.

How many of your favorite foods are Others Group selections? Do you think that this indicates the need for change in your personal food tastes?

STEP 3: THOSE HIGH-FAT FOODS AGAIN

Foods high in fat content usually are guilty of containing more calories than nutrients per serving. And, as you learned on Days Four, Thirteen, and Fourteen, an excessive intake of food fat can result in specific health detriments. To avoid having a high-fat, low-nutrient diet, try to minimize your intake of the following:

bacon
bacon fat
chocolate
cream—heavy, light, sour, whipped
cream cheese
fatty meats
fried foods (vegetables, potatoes, meats, fish, poultry)

Food Likes	Others Group (✔)	High in Fat (✔)	High in Sugar (✔)	High in Salt (✔)	Alcoholic (✔)
Potato chips	✔	✔		✔	

lard
mayonnaise
meat drippings and gravies
olives
pastries and other fatty/fried sweets
salad dressings
salt pork
tartar sauce

Certain high-fat Others Group foods contain appreciable amounts of vitamins and/or minerals, but intake still should be minimized; remember that these foods are high in fat calories:

avocado
butter
margarine
oils (corn, cottonseed, peanut, safflower, sesame, soy, sunflower, walnut)
nuts

It requires both selectivity and willpower to be able to follow a diet which contains only those foods which appeal to the tastebuds, yet still meet nutrient and caloric needs.

STEP 4: SWEET 'n LOW, VERY LOW...

The average American consumes close to one hundred and thirty pounds of refined sugar every year. This means that the average daily intake is equivalent to:

- 40 teaspoons of sugar
- 600 calories from sugar

If you find this hard to believe in your own case, or if you do not consider yourself to have a "sweet tooth," remember that there are considerable amounts of refined sugars hidden in your foods. Refined sugar is present in most processed foods in differing amounts, and appears in various forms:

- table sugar (sucrose)
- corn sugar (corn syrup, corn sweeteners)
- simple sugar (dextrose, glucose, levulose)
- fruit sugar (fructose)
- milk sugar (lactose)
- syrup (honey, maple syrup, molasses)
- "natural" sugar (brown sugar, turbinado sugar, "raw" sugar)

Our bodies do not need any refined sugar. We can obtain all the carbohydrates and calories we need from nutrient-rich starches and natural sugars which are present in fruits, vegetables, grains, and milk products.

Still doubtful that you consume about 40 teaspoons of sugar every day? Consider the following typical day's menu. How many teaspoons of refined sugar do you think it contains?

Breakfast
orange-flavored breakfast drink
granola cereal with milk
toast with grape jelly
coffee with powdered creamer

Mid-morning Coffee Break
glazed donut
coffee with powdered creamer

Lunch
peanut butter and jam sandwich
fruited yogurt
cola

Mid-afternoon Snacks
fudge
chewing gum

Cocktail Hour
whiskey sour
butter-type crackers

Dinner
hamburg-noodle casserole (packaged) with catsup
tossed salad with French dressing
corn niblets (canned)

Dessert
cherry pie or chocolate cake or fig bars or apple-
    sauce or canned fruit or sherbet

Bedtime Snacks
candy bar
cider

Food and Amount From Menu	Approximate Amount of Sugar (in teaspoons)
orange-flavored breakfast drink, ½ cup	4
granola cereal, ¾ cup	1
milk, ½ cup	0
white bread, 2 slices	trace
grape jelly, 1 tbsp	3
coffee, 1 cup	0
powdered creamer, 1 tbsp	1
glazed donut, average size	6
coffee, 1 cup	0
powdered creamer, 1 tbsp	1
white bread, 2 slices	trace
peanut butter, commercial, 2 tbsp	½
strawberry jam, 1 tbsp	3
raspberry yogurt, 1 cup	5
cola, 12 oz can	9
fudge, chocolate, 1 oz	5
chewing gum, 2 sticks	1
whiskey sour (mix), 6 oz	3
butter-type crackers, 10 to 12	1
hamburg, 3 oz	0
noodle mix (packaged), 1 cup	9
catsup, 2 tbsp	1
tossed salad	0
French dressing, 2 tbsp	1
corn niblets, canned, ½ cup	1
cherry pie, average slice	10
chocolate cake, frosted, large slice	10
fig bars, 2	10
applesauce, sweetened, 1 cup	9
canned fruit, with syrup, 1 cup	9
sherbet, 1 cup	9
candy bar, chocolate-covered nougat	5
cider, 1 cup	6

Total Sugar: _____123½_____ teaspoons

So, what is your guess for the amount of sugar in the above menu—a few teaspoons? A cup? More? Now look at the sugar content calculations given here. Note that these are only estimates, useful in illustrating how refined sugar is hidden in our foods. Actual sugar quantities of processed foods differ, depending on the brand.

This is equivalent to an intake of about two and one half cups of sugar—in only one day!

Obviously, it is very easy to consume a large amount of refined sugar without even adding a single teaspoonful at the table. Because so many processed foods contain added sugar, and processed foods now make up a growing proportion of our diets, it is nearly impossible to avoid refined sugar entirely. For most people, this is unnecessary anyway. The key is to be aware of your sugar intake, and thereby consume only a moderate amount.

STEP 5: SWEET TOOTHACHES

Sugar is not poisonous, nor is it a proven health hazard. However, refined sugar merely provides calories with negligible accompanying nutrients. Devoid of nutritional value yet high in caloric con-tent, most sugary foodstuffs are such palate pleasers that we tend to overindulge when we eat them. A diet high in sugar calories, like any high calorie diet, can lead to overweight. And some of the problems associated with excess poundage, such as heart disease, high blood pressure and diabetes, are definite health hazards. Thus, our diets should contain only moderate amounts of any sugar-rich Others Group foods.

A diet high in refined sugar can be detrimental to oral health: a "sweet tooth" is often a decayed one. Dietary carbohydrate serves as the energy source for bacteria which is normally present in the mouth. When allowed to accumulate, this bacteria forms a sticky film called plaque, and an acidic waste is produced. This acid can weaken teeth and result in tooth decay.

Elimination of carbohydrate from the diet, however, is unnecessary and undesirable for optimal nutritional health. Dental decay can be successfully halted by a restricted intake of sticky, sugary, carbohydrate foods. It is the frequent consumption of retentive sweets which tends to increase production time of the undesirable decay-causing acid.

Check (✓) those foods from the following list

which could contribute to the production of dental decay:

____ donuts	____ sweetened yogurt
____ pastry	____ presweetened cereals
____ cookies	____ dried fruit
____ cake	____ fruit in syrup
____ pie	____ table sugar
____ candy	____ brown sugar
____ chewing gum	____ "raw" sugar
____ marshmallows	____ honey
____ sherbet	____ molasses
____ ice cream	____ syrups
____ gelatin, flavored	____ jams, jellies, preserves
____ pudding	____ fruit-flavored drinks
____ custard	____ soft drinks
	____ milkshakes

All of the above foods can contribute to tooth decay. Fluids which contain sugar, however, tend to have a lesser acid-production time because liquids wash through rather than adhere to the teeth. Dietary starches are preferable carbohydrate choices, however, since they usually are lower in decay-causing potential and higher in nutritional value than refined sugars.

STEP 6: WHAT ABOUT FRUCTOSE AND HONEY?

Fructose, a simple sugar found in fruits and honey, is often promoted as the "healthy, natural" alternative to table sugar. Yet, fructose is only as "natural" as refined sugar, since we obtain it from fruits and honey in a manner very similar to that used in processing sugar cane and sugar beet into table sugar.

Fructose is advertised as being much sweeter than sugar, yet the sweetness of fructose depends on the temperature, the degree of acidity, and the concentration. Research has indicated that fructose is indistinguishable from sucrose in hot drinks, cold cereals, and desserts; only in cold, acidic beverages—such as iced tea and lemonade—does fructose taste sweeter than sucrose.

Fructose is also promoted as an alternative sweetener for diabetics, since it causes less dramatic changes in blood sugar levels. Fructose is absorbed more slowly than sucrose, and blood sugar peaks and dips to a lesser extent. However, no long-term well-controlled studies have yet demonstrated significant benefits in the use of fructose by diabetics. Research is still underway.

Honey is often promoted as a high nutrient "superfood." Yet, honey only provides trace amounts of a few vitamins and minerals. Impractically large amounts of honey would have to be consumed in order to obtain any significant nutritional benefits. To illustrate this fact, look at the chart below, which shows the amount of honey one would have to consume in order to obtain the same amount of calcium, iron, and phosphorus provided by other "natural" foods.

Obviously, the fruit sugar provided by honey and other fructose-containing products is about as low in nutritional value as its caloric equivalent, refined sugar.

Remember that sugar is not "bad," nor is it necessary to avoid all foods containing refined sugars. A moderate amount of sugar makes food taste better, and adds enjoyment to eating.

STEP 7: SALT TALK

Sodium is an essential nutrient required by the body for proper functioning (see Day Six). Since sodium is naturally present in most foods, the amount needed each day is easily obtained through a well-balanced diet. However, most Americans tend to consume far more sodium than required through excessive use of salt at the table and in cooking. Most processed foods also contain substantial amounts of sodium in the form of:

- salt—sodium chloride
- MSG—monosodium glutamate
- additives—benzoate of soda, di-sodium phosphate, sodium benzoate, sodium bicarbonate, sodium propionate, sodium saccharin, sodium silico aluminate

A diet high in sodium may contribute to high blood pressure in susceptible individuals. People with high blood pressure have a greater risk of suffering heart attacks, strokes, and kidney disease. The relationship of salt to certain diseases is still under study, but a diet low in sodium may help to prevent high blood pressure, and can aid in treatment when present. If necessary, your physician can prescribe a special low-sodium diet plan.

Nutrient and Amount	Food, and Amount to Obtain Nutrient (Plus calories)	Amount Honey to Obtain Nutrient (Plus calories)
calcium, 296 mg	skim milk, 1 cup (88 calories)	296 tbsp (18,944 calories)
iron, 16.2 mg	liver, 3 oz (234 calories)	162 tbsp (10,368 calories)
phosphorus, 103 mg	egg (82 calories)	103 tbsp (6592 calories)

However, everyone can benefit by avoiding excessively salty foods, and by trying to be moderate in sodium intake.

Does your diet actually contain more sodium than you think? The *Dietary Goals* suggested a moderate daily salt intake of about five grams, or two grams of sodium. A single teaspoon of table salt contains over two grams of sodium. Consider the following typical day's menu. How many grams of sodium do you think it contains? Estimate the number of teaspoons of salt provided by this menu:

Breakfast
tomato juice
fried egg
bacon
corn flakes with milk

Mid-morning Coffee Break
pumpernickel toast with margarine
milk

Lunch
bouillon and crackers
hot dog on buttered roll with catsup, mustard, and relish
dill pickle spears

potato chips
cola

Cocktail Hour
martini
crackers and cheese
peanuts

Supper
Big Mac
tossed salad with Italian dressing
chocolate pudding

Bedtime Snacks
beer
pretzels
peanut butter 'n crax

Now look at the approximate sodium content for the above menu. Note that these are only estimates, as actual sodium contents can vary from item to item.

This is equivalent to an intake of over five teaspoons of table salt—in only one day!

Obviously, it is very easy to consume a large amount of sodium without even shaking your salt shaker. Because so many processed foods contain added sodium, and processed foods now make up

Food and Amount from Above Menu	Approximate Amount of Sodium (in milligrams)
tomato juice, canned, 1 cup	486
egg, fried	155
bacon, 2 slices	306
corn flakes, 1 cup	251
milk, skim, ½ cup	64
pumpernickel bread, 2 slices	364
margarine, 2 tsp	92
milk, skim, ½ cup	64
bouillon, 1 cup	960
crackers, oyster, 20	166
hot dog	627
roll	202
butter, 1 tbsp	140
catsup, 1 tbsp	156
mustard, 2 tsps	126
relish, 1 tbsp	107
dill pickles, 3 spears	1276
potato chips, 1 oz package	191
cola, 12 oz can	54
martini	trace
olives, 2	136
crackers, butter-type, 6	216
cheese, processed American, 2 oz	922
peanuts, ½ cup	301
Big Mac	1510
tossed salad	trace
Italian dressing, 2 tbsp	628
chocolate pudding, 1 cup	335
beer, "light," 2 cans (12 oz each)	112
pretzels, thin, 10	504
peanut butter 'n crax, 2 oz package	592

Total Sodium: __11,043__ milligrams

a growing proportion of our diets, it would be impossible (and unnecessary) to avoid salt entirely. The key is to be aware of your salt intake, and thereby consume only a moderate amount.

STEP 8: SHAKING THE SALT

Since sodium is naturally present in most of our foods, it would be impossible to totally eliminate sodium from the diet. And since sodium is an essential mineral, it would also be undesirable to do so. Instead, sodium intake should be kept to a moderate level by elimination of table salt (at the table and in cooking), and minimal consumption of salty foods. This also requires the following practices:

- careful label reading
- substitution of lemon juice, herbs, and spices for salt
- identification of high-sodium products

You may want to use the following list as a guide in identifying those foods which are especially high in sodium:

Fruit and Vegetable Group
canned vegetables
frozen lima beans, mixed vegetables, peas
pickled beets
pickled salad mix
sauerkraut
seasoned vegetables (frozen)
tomato juice
vegetable juice cocktail

Grain Group
breadsticks (unless unsalted)
crackers (unless unsalted)
popcorn, commercial
pretzels
rolls, salted top

Meat and Alternates Group

bologna	anchovies
chipped beef	canned fish
corned beef	caviar
dried meat	dried fish
frankfurters	herring
ham	sardines
kosher meats	processed cheese
luncheon meats	spread cheese
pastrami	peanut butter
pickled meats	nuts, salted
sausage	
smoked meat or fish	
smoked tongue	
stew, canned	

And Then There's
bacon
bouillon
chips (corn, potato, cheese curls)
dips
olives
soft drinks
soups (canned, frozen, dry package)
condiments: catsup, horseradish, mustard, pickles, relishes, salad dressings, and sauces (barbecue, chili, meat, soy, tartar, Worcestershire)
seasonings: cooking wines, gravies, meat marinades, meat tenderizers, meat/vegetable extracts, monosodium glutamate, salts (celery salt, garlic salt, kosher salt, onion salt, sea salt, seasoned salts)

STEP 9: ADDITIONAL SALT TALK

Herbs and spices can provide a delicious method for decreasing the amount of salt used in food preparations. When used properly, herbs and spices can enliven almost any low-sodium dish, and introduce you to a whole new world of flavors!

pepper	celery seed	rosemary
mustard	tarragon	dill
nutmeg	oregano	savory
cinnamon	sage	marjoram
cloves	parsley	chives
garlic	thyme	

Most Americans only utilize the first seven seasonings, partially due to ignorance, but mostly because of lack of creativity in the kitchen. Perhaps now is the time for you to trade in your salt shaker for some spicy new herbal seasonings!

Herbs

- Fresh herbs are best; flavor can be preserved by freezing in air-tight bags.
- Allow ¼ tsp dried or 1 tsp fresh herbs per pound of meat and per pint of soup or sauce; increase to suit personal tastes.
- When a dish is to be cooked for a long period of time, add herbs during the last hour of cooking.
- For cold dishes, add herbs several hours in advance, or let stand overnight.
- Keep herbs in a cool, dry place—not near the stove—to maintain flavor; keep tightly covered and use within one year.
- Chop or crumble dried leaf herbs before using, to release oils.
- When dish is to be cooked for a short period of time, soak dried herbs for half an hour in a small amount of liquid which is called for in the recipe.

Spices

- Allow ¼ tsp spice per pound (of fruit, meat, etc) or per pint (of sauce, batter, etc).
- Add ground spices at the end of a long-cooking dish.
- Add ground spices to cold dishes several hours before serving.
- Add whole spices at the beginning for a long-cooking dish.
- Crumble or pulverize whole spices to release flavor.
- Heat spiced foods carefully to avoid scorching the spices.
- Store spices like herbs to avoid unnecessary loss of flavor.

Do not be afraid to experiment. Try new seasonings, one at a time or in different combinations. Measure and taste as you prepare, and reseason as needed when you reheat. Lemon juice is another good flavor enhancer, whether bottled or freshly squeezed. Some creative seasoning ideas are given on Days Twenty-One and Twenty-Three.

Note: An overdose of potassium, contained in most salt substitutes, can be dangerous. Use salt substitutes only if prescribed by your physician.

STEP 10: HERE'S TO YOUR HEALTH?

Alcoholic beverages can be a significant source of calories. In fact, alcohol provides 10% to 20% of total caloric intake for the average American. And when alcohol intake interferes with the consumption of nutritious foods, serious nutritional deficiencies can result.

Alcohol is rapidly absorbed from the stomach, although the presence of food will delay this process. Approximately 90% of the alcohol we drink is processed in the liver, and the liver can handle only one liter of alcohol in 24 hours; this means that only ⅔ of an ounce of whiskey or eight ounces of beer can be processed per hour.

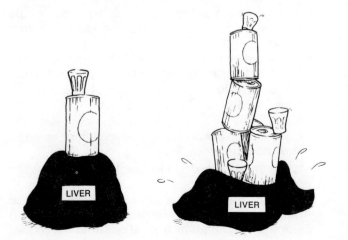

Obviously, the liver cannot meet all the demands made on it by heavy drinkers. As a result, fat deposits form, and liver disease develops. The heart and muscles become wasted, weakened, and filled with fluid. The lining of the stomach can become inflamed, and bleeding will result. Alcohol use can also bring on attacks of gout, and may contribute to low blood sugar. Alcohol abuse during pregnancy can lead to fetal alcohol syndrome, which causes facial, limb, and heart defects.

A moderate intake of alcohol, however, is currently believed to provide some health benefits, perhaps because it encourages relaxation, and thus acts to relieve stress. In amounts not exceeding two to three drinks per day, alcohol intake is associated with the following health benefits:

- lowered blood cholesterol levels (elevated HDLs)
- lowered risk of heart attack
- lowered blood pressure in hypertensive individuals
- improved appetite in elderly persons

The physical and psychological complications associated with alcohol abuse, however, are only too obvious. As usual, moderation is the key.

How many alcoholic beverages do you consume daily? And what types of alcoholic drinks do you usually select? Use your Nutri-Plan diet diary to examine your own drinking habits. In the chart on page 107, list each alcoholic beverage and the amounts consumed since Day One. Total the number of ounces consumed during the two-week period and divide by 14; this will give you your average daily intake in ounces. Does your average daily intake appear to be a moderate amount, or do you need to make some habit changes?

Note also the types of alcoholic beverages you tend to consume: do you drink sweetened mixes, sweet wines, and/or cordials/liqueurs? Do you opt for ales and heavy beers? What are some wiser, low-calorie choices?

STEP 11: ALCOHOL AND CALORIES

Alcohol yields approximately seven calories per gram. (Remember that fat provides nine calories per gram, while both protein and carbohydrate yield four calories per gram.) Alcohol provides few, if any, accompanying nutrients. One pint of bourbon has more than 1200 calories, perhaps the total daily amount your body requires. A single slice of whole wheat bread is far richer in nutrient content than a bottle of beer. Alcohol can provide significant nutritional value only when mixed with a nutritious juice or with milk.

It is easy to overlook the fact that beverages, including alcoholic beverages, can provide calories. The chart on page 107 depicts the approximate caloric worth of several popular alcoholic beverages:

Date—Day:	Alcoholic Beverage and Amount (in ounces)

Total: _____ ounces

Average Daily Intake (÷ 14): _____ ounces

Alcoholic Beverage	Proof	Amount	Calories
liquor, distilled	80	1½ oz	95
liquor, distilled	86	1½ oz	105
liquor, distilled	90	1½ oz	115
liquor, distilled	100	1½ oz	125
liqueur or cordial	60	1 oz	100
beer, "light"	3.2	12 oz	95
beer	4.5	12 oz	150
ale	5	12 oz	165
wine, table	12	3½ oz	90
wine, fortified	19	3½ oz	140
wine, dessert-type	19	3½ oz	150

And a mere six ounces of mixer can add even more calories:

Mixer (6 oz)	Calories
bloody Mary	45
tonic	55
collins	60
ginger ale	60
Seven Up	75
bitter lemon	85
pina colada	285

STEP 12: CALORIES ARE NOT ALL...

In addition to the number of non-nutritious calories they contribute, alcoholic beverages consumed in large amounts tend to diminish the appetite. Consequently, heavy drinkers tend not to eat enough, and often have a highly unbalanced dietary intake. In consideration of the medical complications of alcohol abuse, the importance of maintaining an adequate diet becomes obvious.

Immoderate consumption of alcoholic beverages can lead to a variety of nutritional problems, including:

- dehydration—the body uses about eight ounces of water for the metabolism of each ounce of alcohol consumed; in hot weather, following heavy exercise, or at high altitudes, alcohol intake can result in severe dehydration.
- decreased nutrient absorption—alcohol interferes with the absorption of fats, certain B-vitamins, and the fat-soluble vitamins A, D, and E; vitamin deficiency diseases can result, including anemias and nerve disorders.
- increased nutrient losses—alcohol causes a heightened excretion of certain proteins and minerals; a magnesium deficiency may actually contribute to the symptoms of delirium tremens ("DTs")
- malnutrition—an overall deficiency in important nutrients results in an increased susceptibility to alcohol-induced medical disorders.

Excessive alcohol intake increases the chances for body organ dysfunctions, muscle and nerve damage, and nutritional deficiencies. Extra nutrients are often required in order to correct deficits and to repair any tissue damaged by alcohol excess.

The decision to drink alcohol is personal, usually made early in life, on impulse, and with very little knowledge of possible consequences. Yet, we all need to be aware of the probable ill effects, including the nutritional implications.

Why not try some of the following nutritious alternatives, which contain more nutrients, fewer calories, and are guaranteed to be hangover-free! More nutritious beverage ideas are included on Days Twenty-One and Twenty-Three.

- fresh fruit juices
- fruit juice spritzers (add club soda)
- mineral water
- vegetable juices

If you do choose to include alcoholic beverages in your diet—remember that a moderate intake may provide health benefits—follow these guidelines for safe usage:

- Be moderate in your intake; limit yourself to two or three drinks per day.
- The presence of food in the stomach will help to slow down the rate at which alcohol is absorbed.
- Do not use alcohol with other drugs; alcohol can increase the strength of another drug, even to a fatal degree, or it may destroy drug effectiveness.
- Do not use alcohol if you have a medical conition that warrants temperance.

STEP 13: DAY FIFTEEN PLAN

Continue to record everything you eat and drink in your Nutri-Plan diet diary. For Day Fifteen, continue to be aware of your nutrient intake and to select foods wisely from the basic food groups.

At the end of Day Fifteen, complete the checklist given below and indicate (✔) the behavioral changes you have made. It has now been more than two weeks since you began the Nutri-Plan. You are halfway there!

Halfway Checklist

_____ I do not consume an excessive amount of protein.

_____ I do consume a good amount of carbohydrate in the form of starch.

_____ I do not include too much fat in my diet.

_____ I do eat a variety of vitamin-rich foods.

_____ I do eat a variety of mineral-rich foods.

_____ I do include plenty of water in my diet.

_____ My calorie intake approximates that level which I determined to be desirable for me.

_____ I do obtain the recommended number of daily servings from the basic food groups.

_____ I do consume foods which are high in fiber.

_____ I do try to avoid high-fat and high-cholesterol foods.

_____ I do try to avoids food high in sugar content.

_____ I do try to avoid foods high in salt (sodium) content.

_____ I am moderate in my consumption of alcohol.

_____ My overall diet has improved since Day One.

_____ I consider my diet to be well balanced.

In consideration of the amount of dietary change you may have made so far, it is hard to imagine that even more change is possible. The road to good health is not an easy one, but the end results make the travel worthwhile. And improved health through good nutrition is certainly a destination to strive for.

DAY SIXTEEN

DIETING DOS

STEP 1: THE WEIGH NOT TO GO, OR HOW TO KEEP FAT

If you are overweight and want to remain so, the following guidelines can be of assistance:

- Think about food constantly—daydream about eating rich, high-calorie food stuffs until imagination must become reality.
- Spend a lot of time around food—cook rich, fatty meals, bake desserts and, for goodness sake, taste everything.
- Always shop for food on an empty stomach—everything looks so delicious and appealing when you are hungry that you will tend to buy high-calorie low-nutrient products.
- Keep high-calorie foods on hand—have chips, cookies, and other goodies around the house, in particular near the television, by the phone, in desk drawers, and in the glove compartment of your car.
- Eat when you are not hungry—never bother to wait to eat until you need energy (calories), but instead, eat until you have no energy left for anything else.
- Always "clean your plate"—remember when your parents forced you to eat all you were served "because people are starving in other countries." Well, they will not benefit from anything you leave behind, and if anyone else leaves a bite or two, you eat it.
- Eat hurriedly—your body will not have a chance to notify your brain that you are full, allowing you to eat more and more until you are over-stuffed.
- Concentrate on other activities while eating—watch television, talk on the phone, drive, keep busy, and before you realize it, you will have eaten much more than you had planned.
- Always start your diet "tomorrow"—until "tomorrow" you are free to eat anything and everything; after all, who knows how long you will be dieting, so you may as well have a hot fudge sundae while you still can.
- Be compulsive about food—whenever the urge to eat strikes you, be sure to do so; if you do not feel like stopping when you are overdoing it, keep stuffing yourself.
- Use food as a substitute—eat instead of doing anything else; substitute food for:
  —a good chat with a friend
  —solving a personal problem
  —tackling an unavoidable problem
  —work, fun, sex, socializing
  —facing yourself.

So, go ahead and eat the whole thing. After all, you deserve it, right?

STEP 2: THE WEIGH NOT TO GO, OR FAT FADS

It is estimated that around one third of all Americans are currently overweight. While the exact total is unknown, obesity is one of the most prevalent public health problems. And although millions of dollars are spent each year to try to get rid of the excess poundage, there has been little success in the permanent cure of overweight.

It is probably quite obvious that the following fad diets usually prove to be as unsuccessful as they are unbalanced:

- Starvation diet
- Modified fast
- Grapefruit diet
- Combination foods diet (eg, egg and bananas diet, cottage cheese and fruit diet, etc)
- Beverly Hills diet
- Ice cream diet

- Fruitarian diet (fruit only)
- Drinking man's diet
- Low-carbohydrate diet
- US ski team diet
- Dr Stillman's diet
- Dr Atkin's diet
- I Love New York diet
- Southampton diet
- High-protein diet
- Low-protein diet
- Liquid protein diet
- Cambridge diet
- Liquid diet

Many of these diets may work—temporarily. They can be low enough in caloric content to allot for some loss of body fat, and are low enough in carbohydrate to cause loss of body fluids. Yet, each of these diets—and all fad diets—are adopted by fad dieters with these same expectations:

- I am going to try this diet, and it will be the last diet I will ever have to go on.
- This diet does not include anything I like to eat, so it should work.
- I need to go on this diet for only two weeks, deprive myself for only two short weeks, and then I can eat all the foods I love.
- This diet will be easy: I do not have any choice, and none of the foods will tempt me to overeat.

What is your personal diet history? Consider your own fad diet failures and/or successes, and answer the questions below by checking (✔) the answer for each which best applies to you:

1) In the past, how many fad diets have you tried?
- ☐ 0
- ☐ 1 to 2
- ☐ 3 to 5
- ☐ 6 to 10
- ☐ 11 to 100
- ☐ more than 100

2) In the past, about how many total pounds have you lost through fad diets?
- ☐ 0
- ☐ 1 to 2
- ☐ 3 to 10
- ☐ 11 to 20
- ☐ 21 to 30
- ☐ 31 to 50
- ☐ more than 50

3) Have you kept off any of the lost poundage?
- ☐ Yes
- ☐ No
If so, how many pounds were lost and kept off?
- ☐ 1 to 2
- ☐ 3 to 10
- ☐ 11 to 20
- ☐ 21 to 30
- ☐ 31 to 50
- ☐ more than 50

4) List all fad diets which you have tried in the past: _____
_____
_____
_____

STEP 3: THE WEIGH NOT TO GO, OR DIET PILL-POPPING PROBLEMS

The two basic categories of diet pills are:

- over-the-counter diet aids
- prescription medications

Non-prescription, over-the-counter diet aids are rarely effective and have resulted in several suits for misleading advertisement. These pills contain one or more of the following components:

- Bulk Producers—In combination with liquids, these non-caloric substances fill the stomach to cause a feeling of fullness; unfortunately, appetite is often governed more by the mind than by the belly, and overweight people tend to eat despite feeling physically full.
- Diuretics—Non-prescription "water pills," usually weak and ineffective, stimulate loss of body fluids; once use is halted, these lost fluids return, along with any lost weight—remember that weight loss does not always mean fat loss.
- Phenylpropanolamine Hydrochloride—a mild stimulant, as yet unproven as an effective weight loss agent, this drug is found in products which also provide a limited-calorie diet plan; it is the caloric restriction, rather than a mild "up," which will cause any possible weight loss.
- Benzocaine—related to novocaine, this mild anesthetic supposedly serves to deaden the taste buds and diminish the appetite; again, this drug is yet unproven as an effective weight loss agent, and any resulting loss of weight is usually only temporary.

Reducing candies contain added vitamins and minerals (sometimes bulk producers are added), and supposedly decrease appetite. These expensive candies work on the old premise your parents used to tout: Do not eat candy before your meals, as it will spoil your appetite. Note that a low-calorie diet plan is usually included, since no one can really lose weight simply by adding calories in the form of a candied vitamin supplement.

Prescription diet medications are merely stronger forms of over-the-counter diet aids, offering many unhealthy side effects, yet little success in achieving permanent loss of weight. These pills contain one or more of the following components:

- Amphetamines—causing a physical and psychological "up" with an accompanying lack of appetite, the exact method of function is not clearly understood; although successful for some temporarily, the side effects can prove serious, and include nervousness, shakes, irritability, insomnia, and possible addiction.

• Digitalis—a heart stimulant, it is believed to also stimulate the body to burn fat; unreliable results at a considerable risk to health make this drug an unsafe, ineffective diet aid.

• Thyroid Extracts—thyroid is a hormone which speeds up body rate and may affect body fat storage; again, serious side effects make use undependable and risky.

• Human Chorionic Gonadotropin—HCG is a sex hormone, unproven in affecting weight loss, yet popular in a number of diet clinics; used mainly as a means for charging exorbitant fees, diet clinics using HCG rely on simultaneous caloric restriction to achieve weight losses.

Have you ever tried any of the above diet pills? If so, list them in the chart below, and comment on any accompanying weight losses. Did any of these pills lead to permanent weight loss?

STEP 4: THE WEIGH TO GO

Proper weight control, like a balanced diet, is merely a matter of establishing priorities. If you now have the following characteristics and ideals, you should be able to shed excess poundage quite easily:

• a true desire to lose weight
• the attitude conducive to weight loss
• the patience to adopt a new, lifelong eating pattern
• realistic weight loss goals
• the education required to integrate a well-balanced diet plan into your own lifestyle

If you honestly believe that you need and are ready for a weight loss program, start now:

1) Weigh yourself, and record on the following Nutri-Plan weight chart on page 112. For easy access in the future, post the chart in your bedroom or bathroom.

2) Review your Nutri-Plan diet diary to determine whether you:

• recorded all foods and beverages and the amounts consumed.
• modified your diet from Day One to Day Fifteen.
• adjusted your caloric intake to meet your average daily need.

Diet Pill: Brand Name and Main Ingredient	Length of Time Taken	No. of Pounds Lost	Comments

3) Focus on the food habits illustrated in your Nutri-Plan diet diary in order to determine:

• your own food-related behaviors.
• lifelong food habits which need modification.
• how you can adopt a permanent health-promoting diet plan.

Nutri-Plan Weight Chart

Weigh yourself first thing in the morning, without clothing, once a week. On the chart below, record the date and your weight. Then plot your weight on the graph to assist in better visualization of your weight loss pattern.

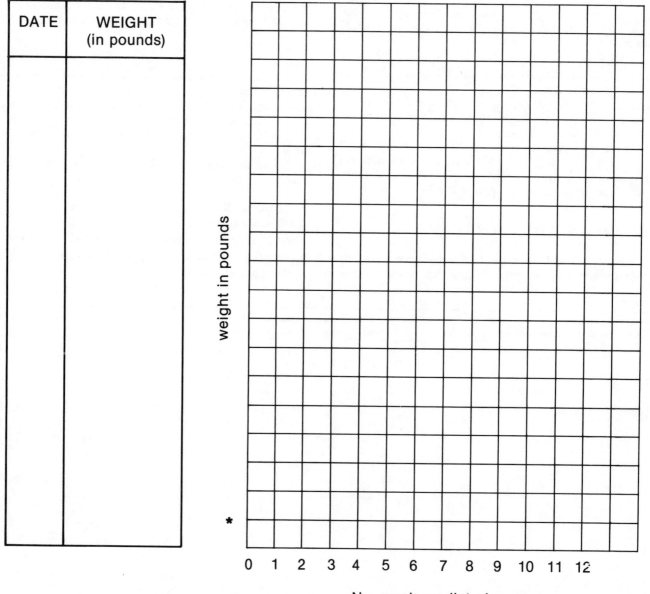

DATE	WEIGHT (in pounds)

weight in pounds

No. week on diet plan

*Ready the graph by filling in your weight goal here, and plotting weights up this axis at two pound increments until reaching your present weight; depending on your individual loss goals, you may not need to plot weights all the way to the top of the graph, or you may require additional plotting space.

STEP 5: STOP COUNTING CALORIES... NUTRI-PLAN DIET PLANS

During the past two weeks, you have begun to try to follow a diet which includes a minimum of the following:

- four servings from the Fruit and Vegetable Group
- four servings from the Grain Group
- two servings from the Milk and Cheese Group (for adults; three servings for children; four for teens)
- two servings from the Meat and Alternates Group

You have also begun to try to be moderate in your intake of foods from the Others Group, and you have been counting calories. You have prob-

ably been thinking that there must be a simpler, faster way to accomplish all of this, so that you have time and energy left to enjoy your food! And there is:

Nutri-Plan Diet Plan

- Choose the Nutri-Plan diet plan which best approximates your average daily caloric intake needs. Remember that a diet including fewer than 1000 calories does not allow for the inclusion of all of the nutrients essential for good health, and tends to be only temporary due to the physical and psychological deprivation it causes.
- By including the allowed daily food group servings in the appropriate serving sizes, you can have a well-balanced diet while remaining within your desired caloric limitations.

Nutri-Plan 1000 Diet Plan
(1000 calories)

Allowed Daily Food Group Servings:
Fruit—2   Milk and Cheese—2   Vegetable—2
Meat and Alternates—4   Grain—4   Fat—3
+ Luxury

Meal Pattern	Sample Menu (with serving equivalents)
Breakfast 1 Grain ½ Milk 1 Fruit	½ cup oatmeal (1 Grain) ½ cup skim milk (½ Milk) 2 tbsp raisins (1 Fruit) coffee, black (unlimited)

Lunch
1 Meat
1 Fat
1 Grain
 	
1 Milk
1 Fruit
	Sandwich:
	    ¼ cup tuna fish (1 Meat)
	    2 tsp low-calorie mayonnaise (1 Fat)
	    2 sl thin-slice wheat bread (1 Grain)
	    lettuce (unlimited)
	1 cup skim milk (1 Milk)
	½ apple, sliced (1 Fruit) sprinkled with cinnamon
	    (unlimited)

Supper
3 Meat
1 Grain
2 Fat
2 Veg
 	
Luxury
	3 oz broiled chicken (3 Meat)
	1 small baked potato (1 Grain)
	2 tbsp sour cream (1 Fat)
	½ cup asparagus, steamed (1 Veg)
	tossed salad:
	    lettuce (unlimited)
	    ½ cup mixed raw veg (1 Veg)
	low-calorie dressing (1 Fat)
	1 av slice sponge cake (Luxury)

Snacks 1 Grain ½ Milk	3 whole rye crackers (1 Grain) ½ cup skim milk (½ Milk)

• Include a variety of foods within each basic food group, in order to ensure the intake of all of the nutrients necessary for health and well-being.

• Avoid the excess calories provided by fatty foods and hidden fats by excluding fried foods, fatty foods, untrimmed meats, high-fat processed foods, gravies and sauces; remember to read the labels and note (*) in your Nutri-Plan diet plan (see below).

• Moderate your intake of foods from the Others Group, and to lessen feelings of diet deprivation, you may include a luxury food each day (luxury foods are listed below). And make sure that your luxury foods are ones that you will really enjoy!

The Nutri-Plan diet plans are given on the following pages, each with allowed daily food group servings, meal pattern, plus a sample menu

Nutri-Plan 1200 Diet Plan
(1200 calories)

Allowed Daily Food Group Servings:
Fruit—4   Milk and Cheese—2   Vegetable—2
Meat and Alternates—5   Grain—5   Fat—3
+ Luxury

Meal Pattern	Sample Menu (with serving equivalents)
Breakfast	
1 Grain	1 cup puffed rice cereal (1 Grain)
½ Milk	½ cup skim milk (½ Milk)
1 Fruit	½ sm banana (1 Fruit)
	coffee, black (unlimited)
Lunch	Sandwich:
1 Meat	1 oz diced chicken (1 Meat)
1 Fat	2 tsp low-calorie mayonnaise (1 Fat)
2 Grain	2 sl oatmeal bread (2 Grain)
	lettuce (unlimited)
1 Milk	1 cup skim milk (1 Milk)
1 Fruit	1 sm orange (1 Fruit)
Supper	
4 Meat	4 oz veal (4 Meat) broiled with
2 Veg	½ cup mushrooms (1 Veg) in
2 Fat	1 tsp vegetable oil (1 Fat)
	tossed salad:
	lettuce (unlimited)
	½ cup mixed raw veg (1 Veg)
	low-calorie dressing (1 Fat)
1 Grain	½ cup brown rice (1 Grain)
1 Fruit	¼ small cantaloupe (1 Fruit)
Luxury	5 gingersnaps (Luxury)
Snacks	
1 Grain	3 cups popcorn (1 Grain)
1 Fruit	Slim Shake:
	½ cup strawberries (1 Fruit)
½ Milk	½ cup skim milk (½ Milk)
	crushed ice (unlimited)

to illustrate how to make food selections within the plan. Serving sizes for each of the basic food groups are also given. Note that one asterisk(*) indicates that the food contains fat equivalent to ½ fat serving; when eating (*) foods, eliminate ½ fat serving from your total allowed daily food group servings. Two asterisk foods (**) contain fat equivalent to one fat serving; when eating (**) foods, eliminate one fat serving from your total allowed daily food group servings. (Does this seem confusing? It may be somewhat difficult to understand at first, but will soon prove to be an easy, fast method to keep track of your fat intake.)

You may want to post your Nutri-Plan diet plan and serving sizes on your refrigerator or kitchen cupboard for easy access during menu planning.

So, start now! You are on your way to optimal health through improved nutrition.

Nutri-Plan 1500 Diet Plan
(1500 calories)

Allowed Daily Food Group Servings:
Fruit—6   Milk and Cheese—2   Vegetable—2
Meat and Alternates—6   Grain—6   Fat—5
+ Luxury

Meal Pattern	Sample Menu (with serving equivalents)
Breakfast 1 Grain ½ Milk 2 Fruit	¾ cup shredded wheat cereal (1 Grain) ½ cup skim milk (½ Milk) ½ banana (1 Fruit) ½ cup orange juice (1 Fruit) coffee, black (unlimited)
Lunch 2 Meat 2 Fat 1 Milk 2 Grain 2 Fruit	Sandwich: 2 oz boiled ham (2 Meat + 1 Fat) 1½ oz part-skim mozzarella cheese (1 Milk + 1 Fat) mustard (unlimited) 2 sl whole rye bread (2 Grain) lettuce (unlimited) 1 fresh pear (2 Fruit)
Supper 4 Meat 3 Fat 2 Veg 2 Grain 1 Fruit Luxury	4 oz (1 oz each) lean meatballs (4 Meat + 2 Fat) ½ cup tomato sauce (1 Veg + 1 Fat) 1 cup whole wheat spaghetti (2 Grain) Italian salad: lettuce (unlimited) ¼ cup sliced tomatoes (½ Veg) ¼ cup cold green beans (½ Veg) Lemon and vinegar (unlimited) 10 to 12 fresh cherries (1 Fruit) 1 av slice angel food cake (Luxury)
Snacks 1 Grain 1 Fruit ½ Milk	½ whole wheat English muffin (1 Grain) with ½ apple, sliced (1 Fruit) sprinkled with cinnamon (unlimited) ½ cup skim milk (½ Milk)

Serving Sizes

Fruit

10 to 12	cherries, grapes
3	kumquats
2	apricots, dates, passion fruit, plums, prunes
2 oz	guava, quince
1	fig, nectarine, orange, peach, persimmon, tangelo, tangerine
1 cup	casaba melon, watermelon
2 tbsp	raisins
¾ cup	cranberries, currants, strawberries
½ small	apple, banana, grapefruit, mango, papaw, papaya, pear
½ cup	applesauce, berries (black, blue, boysen, logan, rasp), fruit cocktail, pineapple
½ cup juice	grapefruit, orange
⅓ cup juice	apple, cider, nectars, pineapple
¼ cup juice	cranberry, grape, prune
¼ small	cantaloupe, honeydew

Vegetable

½ cup	vegetable juices, all vegetables (except those included in grain group)

Note: All fruits and vegetables should be fresh, frozen, or canned without added sugar or sauces.

Grain

1 slice	bread (all types)
2 slices	thin-sliced bread
½	bagel, bun, English muffin, matzoth
½" square	cornbread
1 small**	biscuit, muffin, pancake, waffle
1 small	mini pita pocket, potato, roll, sweet potato, yam
½ cup cooked	corn, grits, hot cereal, lima beans, pasta, peas, rice, winter squash
¾ cup	dry cereal
1 cup	puffed cereal
¼ cup**	granola
3 cups	popcorn
3	crackers (arrowroot, melba, rye, soda, wheat)
6	saltines
9" diameter	tortilla
¾ oz	buckwheat, millet
2 tbsp	barley (uncooked)
1 tbsp	cracked wheat, wheat berries
¼ cup	bulgur, flour
⅙ cup	breadcrumbs, cornmeal, whole-wheat flour

Milk and Cheese

1 cup	skim milk
1 cup*	low-fat yogurt (plain)
1 oz**	cheese (whole milk)
1½ oz*	cheese (part-skim or skim)

Serving Sizes *(Continued)*

Meat and Alternates

1 oz cooked	chicken, fish, lamb, shellfish, turkey, veal
1 oz cooked*	lean beef, lean pork, organ meats
1 oz cooked**	beef, cold cuts, duck, frankfurter, ham
1	egg
¼ cup	canned fish, dried beans, dried peas, lentils, low-fat cottage cheese
¼ cup*	creamed cottage cheese

Note: Meat should be trimmed of all visible fat, and baked, boiled, broiled, or roasted without added fat. Fish should be canned in water.

Fat

1 strip	bacon
1 tsp	butter, margarine, mayonnaise, oil, peanut butter
2 tsp	cheese/Italian dressing, low-calorie margarine, low-calorie mayonnaise
1 tbsp	cream cheese, French dressing, heavy cream, tartar sauce
2 tbsp	light cream, sour cream
3 tbsp	dry cocoa powder, half-and-half creamer, non-dairy creamer
10	almonds, peanuts
20	pistachios
5 to 6	other nuts, olives

Note: Bacon, nuts, and peanut butter do contain some protein as well.

Luxury

1 oz	liquor
1 av slice	angel food cake, sponge cake
1**	donut (plain)
3	graham crackers
3½ oz	dry wine
5 small	gingersnaps, vanilla wafers
8**	French fries
12 oz	"light" beer
¼ cup	gelatin, sherbet
½ cup**	ice cream (plain)

Note: Luxury foods are rich in fat, sugar, salt, and/or alcohol and are to be eaten only in the moderate amounts outlined in the Nutri-Plan diet plans. You may want to substitute a 75-calorie food choice from another basic food group, or 75 calories of your own special luxury food instead.

Unlimited	bouillon, club soda, coffee, diet soft drinks, herbs, horseradish, lemon, lettuce, lime, low-calorie gelatin, mustard, pickles (sour or dill), radishes, spices, sugar-free gum, tea, vinegar

Note: If you are limiting your intake of sodium, caffeine and/or saccharin, be aware that many of the unlimited items are significant sources of these substances.

---

*Omit ½ fat from total allowed daily food group servings.
**Omit 1 fat from total allowed daily food group servings.

STEP 6: DAY SIXTEEN PLAN

Continue to record everything you eat and drink in your Nutri-Plan diet diary. For Day Sixteen, continue to be aware of your nutrient intake and to select foods wisely from the basic food groups.

At the end of Day Sixteen, use your Nutri-Plan diet diary and the information given in Step 5 in order to total your daily food group servings. In the chart below, list all foods and beverages consumed on Day Sixteen and the amounts. Convert these amounts into daily food group servings and determine the approximate number of servings eaten. Total your daily food group servings for each food group. A sample meal has been illustrated below.

Did you include the allowed daily food group servings appropriate for your individual Nutri-Plan diet plan? Without counting calories, you can easily balance your diet, and remain within your caloric budget as well.

Sample Chart

Food and Amount	Daily Food Group and No. Servings Eaten
orange juice, 1 cup	Fruit—2
rye toast, 1 slice	Grain—1
margarine, 1 tsp	Fat—1
skim milk, ½ cup	Milk—½

Day Sixteen

Food and Amount	Daily Food Group and No. Servings Eaten

Daily Food Group Servings—Totals: Fruit _____
Vegetable _____
Grain _____
Milk and Cheese _____
Meat and Alternatives _____
Fat _____
Luxury _____

DAY SEVENTEEN
MAKING MODIFICATIONS

STEP 1: ORAL ABUSE

There are three common forms of self-abuse which can result in documented, well-known health damages. These three so-called oral abuses with which we tend to inflict ourselves are:

- cigarette smoking
- excessive alcohol consumption
- overeating

A compulsion is an uncontrollable psychological drive to indulge in a particular activity, often abusive. If eating becomes a compulsion, just as with smoking cigarettes and drinking alcohol, the oral abuser feels compelled to overindulge. Unlike smoking and drinking, however, the overeater cannot stop "cold turkey," although this might prove easier for those to whom a single taste inevitably leads to a binge.

Overeating on occasion certainly is not seriously abusive. Many people are unaware of what food represents to them and of how they use food. It is this lack of insight which may have unhealthy results. We all need to learn how to use insight, so that we can begin to develop an increased aware-ness of our personal food habits and eating behaviors.

During the past sixteen days, you have been observing and recording some of your own food-related behaviors. You should now be able to utilize the information presented on Day Seventeen to determine some of the reasons behind your own particular behaviors.

Determining why we do what we do is a complex process, but even a small degree of insight can be of great assistance in achieving self-improvement.

From infancy on, we all develop specific habits and shape our personal views. Eating patterns are also greatly influenced by today's world. And every individual has personal feelings about the emotional aspects of eating, the meaning of food, and the psychological implications of diets. What are your feelings concerning eating, food, and diet? Why do you eat the way you do?

Try to use honest insight in answering the following questions. You may want to refer to your Nutri-Plan diet diary for assistance.

Often	Occasionally	Never	
☐	☐	☐	1) Do you reward yourself with food?
☐	☐	☐	2) Do you feel guilty if you do not eat all of the food which you have been served?
☐	☐	☐	3) Do you associate people, places, and events from the past with specific foods?
☐	☐	☐	4) Does the sight of food make you feel hungry?
☐	☐	☐	5) Does the smell of food make you feel hungry?
☐	☐	☐	6) Does the thought of eating make you feel hungry?
☐	☐	☐	7) Do you eat according to the clock (eg, noontime automatically signifies lunchtime)?
☐	☐	☐	8) Do you eat while simultaneously engaged in other activities (eg, reading, watching television, working—job, house, school —talking on the phone, driving, etc)?
☐	☐	☐	9) Do you eat when you are emotionally stimulated (eg, you turn to food when you are bored, frustrated, nervous, lonely, fatigued, depressed, happy, etc)?
☐	☐	☐	10) Do you put off or avoid unpleasant activities by eating instead?
☐	☐	☐	11) Do you eat because of the influence of others (employer, family, spouse, parents, friends, etc)?
☐	☐	☐	12) Do you find yourself searching unsuccessfully for foods to satisfy unknown cravings?

STEP 2: INFLUENCES FROM THE PAST

As individuals, we all develop different eating behaviors, partially due to our varied pasts. Our own special food habits become instilled in us during infancy, childhood, the teenage years, and early adulthood. Parental influences are also integral to the development of our food-related behaviors.

1) Do you reward yourself with food? Do you turn to food if:

• you have had a particularly difficult day?
• your children were especially troublesome?
• you are not feeling physically up to par?

Or, do you reach for "goodies" whenever you:

• have been dieting successfully for awhile (be it 12 hours, 12 weeks, or 12 months)?
• pass an examination?
• receive a promotion?

Can you remember your parents using food as a reward if you:

• received good grades?
• went to bed when told?
• stopped crying?

Do you reward others with food:

• for good behavior?
• if they have had a difficult day?
• if they are ill or hurt?
• if they meet your demands?
• so that they will love and appreciate you?
• because you consider food to be a just reward?

In all of these situations, food is not used as a means for appeasing physical hunger, but as a way to get or give a psychological lift. Using food to reward yourself or others results in new meanings for food, and develops into a psychological association between feeling good and eating food.

2) Do you feel guilty if you do not eat all of the food which you have been served? If, as a child, you were forced to eat everything on your plate, perhaps even punished if you refused, then you may still feel compelled to "clean the plate." Do you find that you:

• never leave behind the last bite of your meal?
• force others to finish their food?
• allow yourself or others to eat dessert only if the entire meal was consumed?
• eat leftovers from others' plates, rather than have them "wasted"?

Upon serious consideration, doesn't it actually appear more wasteful to overindulge to the point of uncomfortable fullness, than to throw out a mouthful of meatloaf or a bowlful of leftover mashed potato?

3) Do you associate people, places, and events from the past with specific foods? In other words, does:

• hot soup always remind you of being comforted by a loved one when you were cold or ill?
• a trip to the coastline always mean a seafood dinner?
• a sporting event require peanuts and beer?
• dinner's end inevitably mean that dessert shall begin?

Again, food can easily mean much more to us than a way to halt physical hunger. Yet, must we allow our past influences to continue to determine our present eating behaviors? In order that you may begin to exert control over the influences your past may have on your current eating behaviors, try to incorporate the following suggestions into your own lifestyle:

• Choose desirable alternatives to food for use as a reward. For example, reward yourself with a hot, luxurious bath after a difficult day, or reward your husband for his promotion with tickets to a popular play.
• Leave one bite on your plate at each meal or snack—resist the temptation to "clean the plate"; also, avoid the urge to encourage others to eat against their will.
• Whenever you are eating, ask yourself if it is by your own choice, or triggered by someone, someplace, or some event from your past. For example, do you really want to eat chocolate bars on October 31 of every year?

STEP 3: ENVIRONMENTAL INFLUENCES

Eating behaviors are highly susceptible to outside influences. There exists a multitude of cues in the world around us, triggering our psyches and affecting our eating behaviors. Many people learn to respond only to those environmentally-induced, external cues to eat, rather than to their own feelings of physical, internal hunger. Think about what hunger actually feels like to you, and consider its physical symptoms.

4) Does the sight of food make you feel hungry? Is it common for you to:

• run to the kitchen for a snack after viewing a television commercial showing freshly baked chocolate chip cookies?

- drool over the thought of fudge whirl ice cream after seeing signs outside an ice cream parlor?
- feel parched and thirsty whenever you glimpse a billboard promoting beer?
- make a special trip to the local bakery after seeing an inviting magazine photograph of fresh muffins?

Whenever you eat in response to the sight of food, rather than to physical hunger, you are responding falsely. You are allowing your environment to manipulate your eating behaviors and to make food choices for you.

5) Does the smell of food make you feel hungry? For example, is it true that:

- when you are cooking a roast, your nose tempts you into nibbling?
- when you are passing a bakery, the aroma of freshly baked bread draws you inside?
- you never pass up a bucket of popcorn at the movie theater, once the distinct odor reaches your keen nostrils?
- once the aroma of newly baked chocolate chip cookies fills the kitchen, your name becomes "Cookie Monster"?

Again, if allowed to, the environment can direct your eating behaviors. To eat or not to eat, that is the question... the choice should be your own.

6) Does the thought of eating make you feel hungry? Does the idea of indulging in delicious foods preoccupy your thoughts? Do you find yourself:

- fantasizing over hot fudge sundaes whenever you are trying to lose weight?
- fantasizing over chips and cola whenever you are attempting to follow a healthy diet plan?
- concentrating on lunch before breakfast has been finished?
- thinking about food more than anything else?

And when your thoughts turn to food, do they control your mind until you feel that you can halt the torturous process only by eating? Quite often, external cues can cause your mind to get locked in the refrigerator! Do not let your environment put you in the deep freeze. You can control your thoughts, rather than allowing them to control you.

7) Do you eat according to the clock? In other words is:

- noon a four-letter word for lunch?
- six o'clock an automatic alarm which signals the cocktail hour?
- bedtime really snacktime?

- a coffee break simply not the same without coffee —and donuts?

When you eat in response to time, rather than to physical hunger, you are responding to the external and ignoring the internal. Many people become so scheduled in their eating patterns that they actually lose the capacity to interpret their own internal hunger signals.

8) Do you eat while simultaneously engaged in other activities? Are you always eating while doing something else? For example, do you:

- eat your eggs while you skim the morning paper?
- munch, munch, munch in front of the television set?
- polish off leftover chocolates while you polish the silverware?
- have a long phone cord which can be stretched at least as far as your refrigerator?
- keep plenty of "goodies" in the glove compartment of your car?

Oftentimes, if the mind is occupied with an activity, a simultaneous activity is not able to be completely registered. This is the reason why you may find that you have eaten an entire box of popcorn during a movie without even realizing it. It sometimes seems as if someone else has eaten your food! If you do not concentrate on eating as a sole activity, you may not derive all of the associated psychological benefits. Thus, you may find yourself, consciously or unconsciously, eating more than you think, need, or want to eat.

Avoid allowing the environment to maintain control over your eating behaviors. Whenever you begin to eat anything, ask yourself the questions listed below. Each time your response is Yes, recognize the fact that you are eating in response to environmental cues, rather than to a physical need for food. Thus, every time you answer Yes to these questions, you should realize that you have allowed your environment to control you. It is up to you to change your eating behaviors, to be able to say No to these questions and to environmental triggers to eat. Only you can control your environment, your food habits, yourself.

Yes	No	
☐	☐	Did the sight of food cue me to eat, even though I am not physically hungry?
☐	☐	Did the smell of food cue me to eat, even though I am not physically hungry?
☐	☐	Did the thought of eating cue me to eat, even though I am not physically hungry?

Yes No

☐ ☐ Did I allow something in my environment to trigger my hungry mind into fantasizing about food?

☐ ☐ Am I eating only because it is "time to eat"?

☐ ☐ Am I simultaneously involved in another activity while eating?

STEP 4: EMOTIONAL INFLUENCES

Every individual has a variety of personal feelings about food. Foods represent different things to different people, and influence people in many different ways. We eat food for a number of reasons, and it is the responsibility of each individual to determine these reasons. Once you understand why you eat as you do, you may then begin to modify your undesirable food habits.

9) Do you eat when you are emotionally stimulated? For example, whenever:

• bored, creating (and eating) a sandwich provides you with something interesting to do?

• family frustrations have you down, a few cookies will lift your sagging spirits.

• traffic is nerve-racking, a candy bar from the glove compartment calms you down.

• Saturday night is dateless, a bag of chips and a good TV-movie are friends indeed.

Do you sleep with your nightcap, cry into your soup, and rejoice with a hot fudge sundae? Food can serve many important emotional functions, including:

• relief from boredom
• ease of frustration
• soothing of tense nerves
• provision of friendship
• erasure of fatigue
• cheering of woes and enhancement of good cheer.

Yet, food can serve these functions only temporarily. Food is not a cure, but merely a means for delay in dealing with emotional and personal problems. You will not solve your marital problems with a pizza, nor dissolve your financial woes in a chocolate milkshake. In fact, people often end up increasing the severity of their personal problems by choosing to eat, rather than dealing with the issues at hand.

10) Do you put off or avoid unpleasant activities by eating instead? Do you:

• opt for a visit to the local ice cream parlor in favor of a visit to an elderly relative?

• take several extra long coffee (and donut) breaks during a dull or difficult day at the office?

• put off making that dreaded phone call by making (and eating) a sandwich instead?

• prefer tackling hamburgers at the local hangout to tackling homework in your room?

Food can be an excellent substitute for less pleasurable tasks, and eating can serve as an enjoyable, if only temporary diversion. Food can easily be used to avoid confrontation, to escape from duties, even to avoid confronting yourself.

11) Do you eat because of the influence of others? Do your emotions concerning people close to you affect your eating behaviors? For example, does/do:

• your employer drive you to drink?

• your children drive you to date-nut cookies?

• your husband drive you to donuts?

• your parents drive you to cookies and donuts?

Do you find that you always overindulge with your fat friend Edie? Or with your thin neighbor Eddie? Do the "girls" always serve coffee and Danish, and the "boys" always hand around beer and ham sandwiches? Does a broken heart invariably lead to a broken diet? People trigger emotions, and feelings certainly influence eating habits. By determining who stimulates which eating responses, it is possible to learn how to gain control. After all, just because other people are unable to control themselves around us, does not mean that this should have to influence our control over ourselves!

12) Do you find yourself searching unsuccessfully for foods to satisfy unknown cravings? For example, do you find yourself:

• consuming three dill pickles, two tossed salads, one pint of cottage cheese, 12 melba toasts, an apple, a banana, and a "light" beer...before you decide that what you really craved was to dine out?

• gobbling down four different kinds of candy bars, yet still feeling dissatisfied?

• eating an onion omelette while craving attention?

• with your head in the refrigerator, your hand in the cookie jar, and your fingers in a box of chocolates...without any idea of what you are searching for?

It is important to be able to determine the reasons why we want to eat and what our needs are, so that we can successfully satisfy those needs. Insight and self-awareness can affect our choices for undergoing dissatisfying binges or actually dealing with personal problems.

In order that you may begin to exert control over the influences your emotions may have on your eating behaviors, try to incorporate the following suggestions into your own lifestyle:

• Select alternative outlets for emotions and avoid the kitchen when your emotions are stirred. Get a dart board, a close friend, a psychiatrist, or go for a brisk walk when problems arise—and work them out, if possible.

• Whenever tempted to eat instead of undertaking a necessary task, ask yourself, "Will I simply delay the undesirable activity or avoid it altogether if I eat?" Then either do the task or don't; eating is not going to help either way.

• Avoid running to the kitchen whenever others stir up your emotions. Instead, develop alternate places to seek refuge, such as a local park, movie theater, or zoo. It is amazing how much insight can be gained during a few hours of absence from a problem person.

• Before embarking on a frustrating safari in search of that soul-satisfying-something to devour, stop and reflect. By taking some time to determine what your needs are, you can then identify what would satisfy that need. You may even choose not to eat at all!

STEP 5: MODIFYING BEHAVIOR

It is essential that you think of your diet plan as a permanent lifestyle change, rather than as a temporary inconvenience. The results of any successful dieting endeavor can rapidly be erased by a return to old eating habits. Only those diets which modify behavior so that permanent changes in eating habits are made have demonstrated long-term success.

Permanent change appears to be a difficult task, much more demanding than temporary day/week/ month-long fad diets. Yet, it is also obvious why over ninety percent of those who do lose weight simply gain it back—often adding on even more poundage in the process.

The adoption of new habits can assist in the destruction of old habits. And you have been doing just this, gradually, since Day One. You may have noticed that it has been getting successively less difficult each day for you to incorporate new dietary habits. This process will become even easier as you develop clearer insight into your own eating behaviors.

For Day Seventeen, make an especially careful appraisal of your eating behaviors in order to identify those changes you want to make. The following guidelines can assist you in making any necessary dietary modifications:

• Use your Nutri-Plan diet diary and the suggestions given in Steps 2 to 4 to assist you in observing your eating behaviors and developing food habit awareness.

• Determine the influences—past, environmental, emotional—that control your eating behaviors.

• Modify your behaviors as suggested in Steps 2 to 4 in order to encourage new behaviors.

• Develop a new set of eating behaviors to replace your undesirable food habits.

• Focus on strengthening these new eating behaviors.

• Make slow, small changes, and practice new behaviors until they become habitual.

• Take responsibility for yourself and for your lifestyle.

• Do not give up! It takes time and effort to be the person you want to be, but it is well worth it.

STEP 6: DAY SEVENTEEN PLAN

Continue to record everything you eat and drink in your Nutri-Plan diet diary. For Day Seventeen, consider the following suggestions for gaining further insight into and modifying appropriately your personal eating behaviors, and complete the following questionnaire.

1) Choose desirable alternatives to food for use as a reward. List some examples: _____
_____

2) Leave one bite on your plate at each meal or snack—resist the temptation to "clean the plate." Are you successful at this exercise? ☐ Yes ☐ No ☐ Sometimes Why or why not? _____
_____

3) Whenever you are eating, ask yourself if it is by your own choice or triggered by someone, someplace, or some event from your past. Briefly describe some of your conclusions: _____
_____

4) Try not to eat in response to the sight of food; if you do so, briefly describe the event(s) and your feelings at the time: _____
_____

5) Try not to eat in response to the smell of food; if you do so, briefly describe the event(s) and your feelings at the time: _____
_____
_____

6) Avoid fantasizing about food; if you do find yourself fantasizing, briefly explain what you feel may have triggered your thoughts: _____
_____

7) Avoid eating according to the clock; if you are unsuccessful, list some examples of and possible reasons behind your failure(s): _____

_____

_____

8) Avoid eating while engaged in other acitivites by making eating a sole experience. You can note. your success in your Nutri-Plan diet diary.

9) Select alternative outlets for emotions. List some examples: _____

_____

_____

10) Avoid eating for the purpose of procrastination. When you must face an unpleasant task, do you usually: ☐ put it off? ☐ tackle the problem? ☐ eat instead? List some examples: _____

_____

_____

11) Develop places other than the kitchen where you can seek refuge from people who stir up your food-related emotions to an undesirable degree. List some of the places you may choose to utilize:

_____

_____

_____

12) Avoid dissatisfying searches for unknown foods. Whenever you are looking for a specific food to satisfy a particular craving, stop and reflect. List your needs at this time: _____

_____

_____

Are any of these needs edible? If not, do you really need to eat? ☐ Yes ☐ No Describe your feelings on this: _____

_____

_____

DAY EIGHTEEN

NUTRITION—AT HOME

STEP 1: YOUR POA

Select the expression from the choices below that you think POA stands for. Do you have a POA regarding your diet? Do you think you need one?

☐ Party-On Attitude
☐ Pig-Out Allowance
☐ Powerful Oral Abuse
☐ Plan Of Action

In order to effectively execute permanent modifications in lifestyle, a distinct plan of action should be followed. The steps toward the adoption of a lifelong program of healthy eating habits have been outlined day-by-day during the past seventeen days. In order to successfully incorporate the suggested dietary changes, it becomes essential to plan for your future.

In reviewing your Nutri-Plan diet diary, you may notice that you did not always adhere to your intended dietary intake plans. Quite often it is not until after the fact that we realize our mistakes. The best method for avoiding unplanned errors is to get into the habit of planning ahead. By planning out each day's meals and snacks in advance, you are able to ensure that your diet plan meets all of the desired criteria:

- appropriate calorie level for your individual Nutri-Plan diet plan.
- desired number of servings from each of the daily food group servings.
- adequate (but not excessive) serving amounts for all food and beverage selections.
- varied food choices with desirable nutrient contents.

Thus, planning ahead can assist you in the adoption of a well-balanced diet plan appropriate for your own needs and desires. And the best time and place for you to start?

- Right now
- At home
- Let's go!

Begin by asking yourself the following questions; you may want to refer to your Nutri-Plan diet diary (especially comments and personal feelings) in order to take a close look at your home life eating habits:

Yes No

☐ ☐ Does your home environment hinder the incorporation of a well-balanced diet plan (eg, tempting foods all around the house, lack of kitchen facilities, etc)? If Yes, explain: _____
_____
_____

☐ ☐ Does your particular role in the home make dietary change difficult (eg, always cooking or serving tempting foods, family members not helpful in the kitchen, etc)? If Yes, explain: ____
_____
_____

☐ ☐ Do you handle your diet plan and eating patterns differently at home than in other places (eg, only follow diet successfully at home, cannot adhere to diet when home, etc)? If Yes, explain: _____
_____
_____

You now need to develop your own personal POA, one which successfully combines your Nutri-Plan diet plan, your home life, and all other aspects of your individual lifestyle.

STEP 2: HOME IMPROVEMENTS

Do you think that your home environment induces undesirable eating patterns? Complete the following questionnaire about your home:

---

1) Go into the kitchen. List all foods which are easily visible: _____
_____
_____

2) List the changes you could make in your kitchen to reduce or eliminate the visual eating cues (eg, keep baked goods out of sight in the bread drawer): _____
_____
_____

3) List activities normally conducted in your kitchen which can stimulate eating responses (eg, doing homework, talking on the phone, haggling with children): _____
_____
_____

4) List the changes you could make in your kitchen to reduce or eliminate these eating cues (eg, remove desk from kitchen, put or use phone in another room, make kitchen off-bounds for arguments): _____
_____
_____

5) List all other areas of your home where food is readily available (eg, television room, bar, utility room, etc): _____
_____
_____

6) List activities normally conducted in these other areas which can stimulate eating responses (eg, in television room: snack while watching television, playing cards, reading): _____
_____
_____

7) What is the most obvious solution to this problem (of eating in these other areas while simultaneously engaged in alternate activities)?
☐ Board up all rooms which can stimulate eating responses.
☐ Sell your house and start over.
☐ Remove all food from these areas.

The above questionnaire should have provided you with several ideas for home improvements. Utilize the following suggestions as well, so that you may create a home environment which is supportive of your Nutri-Plan diet plan and the dietary changes it entails.

Homely Tips

• Keep all food in the kitchen, and out of sight. Store bread and baked goods in the bread box, fruit in the refrigerator, and snacks in the cabinets, rather than on counters or tables where they are within easy-spying and easy-grabbing distance.

• Store foods in opaque containers and freeze all leftovers to further reduce visual cues.

• Prepare and keep on hand only those foods allowed in your Nutri-Plan diet plan; avoid purchase of tempting high-calorie, low-nutrient foods —out-of-sight may mean out-of-mouth.

• Utilize the kitchen only for eating and food preparation; discourage lingering in the kitchen by removing non-food items such as the television, phone, and all desk/home/office work.

• Avoid entering the kitchen when emotionally upset and vulnerable to food bingeing.

• Remove all food from areas other than the

kitchen; after all, if you do not have any snacks in the television room, and no television in the kitchen, you may have to change your TV-snacking behaviors!

STEP 3: PLANNED EATING PLACE

Where do you conduct most of your unplanned —and often regretted—eating? Do you often find yourself:

- standing at the kitchen sink, cookies in hand?
- munching at the refrigerator door, looking for more?
- wandering around the house, leaving a trail of crumbs behind?
- nibbling while at the stove, in front of the television, or driving in your car?

A planned eating place may assist you in avoiding unplanned overeating. Choose a particular place where you will habitually eat whenever you eat at home. Make sure it has comfortable seating, and does not expose you to eating cues. Snacktime or mealtime, get into the habit of always eating in this particular place, your planned eating place.

Now, complete the following questionnaire on your planned eating place:

- Use small plates to create an image of large serving sizes.
- To lessen the desire for extra helpings, keep serving dishes away from your personal eating place.
- Whenever you are at your personal eating place, avoid other activities, concentrate on your food, and make eating the sole activity.
- Remember to leave that last bite on your plate, and to avoid nibbling food from others' plates.
- If cooking and cleaning up after meals and snacks inevitably stimulates nibbling, have other family members assist you, if possible; your particular role in the home can be adjusted to suit your individual diet and health goals.

Note: Suggestions to assist you when eating away from home are included on Day Twenty.

STEP 4: SERVING SIZE ACCURACY

Portion control is essential when calorie intake is restricted. In order to be sure that you are meeting your Nutri-Plan diet plan daily calorie allotment, your serving sizes from the allowed daily food group servings must be accurate. Until you become adept at judging quantities simply by looking, you

---

1) Describe your planned eating place: _____
_____

2) Is the seating comfortable? Yes ☐ No ☐ Will you be able to eat in a relaxed manner here? Yes ☐ No ☐

3) Are there any visual eating cues present? Yes ☐ No ☐ If Yes, list them: _____
_____
_____

4) Approximate the average daily number of meals and snacks you will eat at your personal eating place: ☐1 ☐2 ☐3 ☐4 ☐5 ☐6 or more.

Utilize the following suggestions, so that you may transform your personal eating place into an environment which is supportive of your Nutri-Plan diet plan and the related behavioral changes.

More Homely Tips

- Eat slowly so that both your body and your psyche will be satisfied with smaller amounts.
- Chew food thoroughly.
- Relax during meals and take time out from eating to chat or rest.

should rely on measuring cups, measuring spoons, and food scales to ensure accuracy. Try the following activity in order to further illustrate this concept:

1) Take each of the items listed in the chart on page 130 and estimate the given amounts (Amount to Estimate) into a glass, bowl, or plate. You may want to substitute similar foods that you have on hand for some of the listed items.
2) Weigh or measure each estimated item. How accurate were you able to be? Did you tend to overestimate or underestimate the actual amounts?

Food	Amount to Estimate	Measured Amount
apple juice	⅓ cup	
strawberries	¾ cup	
asparagus spears	½ cup	
cabbage, chopped	1 cup	
puffed wheat cereal	1 cup	
brown rice	½ cup	
milk, skim	8 oz	
cheese, part-skim	1½ oz	
hamburger	3 oz	
tuna	¼ cup	
butter or margarine	1 tsp	
Italian salad dressing	2 tsp	
beer, "light"	12 oz	
wine, dry	3½ oz	
liquor	1 oz	
soft drink	8 oz	

If you determine through the above exercise that it would be a wise idea for you to measure your food intake until you become more adept at judging serving sizes, try these suggestions to ease the measuring process:

- Keep measuring cups, measuring spoons, and scales visible and within easy reach.
- To become adept at eye-appraisal, measure out serving sizes for all foods and memorize the appearance of each in your glasses, bowls, and on your plates.
- Diet scales can be purchased at your local drug store or supermarket; postal scales tend to provide more accurate results.
- Weigh foods after cooking. To become adept at eye-appraisal of serving sizes, study the appearance of each weighed item.

The chart below illustrates the fact that only a small amount of excess food each day can gradually add up, resulting in unwanted poundage. If you consumed each day, in addition to your caloric needs, any one of the listed foods in the given amounts, you could conceivably gain the indicated number of pounds in just one year. Obviously, skill and accuracy in judging serving sizes is an important aspect of calorie control.

Extra Food and Amount	No. Pounds Gained Per Year
orange, 1 med	5
beer, "light," 6 oz	5
margarine, 1 tsp	5
potato chips, 10	10
fudge, 1 oz	10
chocolate chip cookie, large	10
donut, plain	15
ice cream, plain, 1 cup	30
steak, T-bone, 4 oz	40

STEP 5: FANTASY FOR FUN AND FAT-FIGHTING

Constructive use of imagery can assist in control over behavior. In fact, you can use your imagination to help you in modifying your own eating behaviors. Try the fantasies given below, or devise your own. But first, create the proper atmosphere:

- Relax in a comfortable chair in a calm, quiet environment.
- Close your eyes, and imagine that you are looking at a large, blank television screen.
- Whenever temptation or emotional upheavals occur, project the fantasy of your choice onto your own inner television screen.

In practicing the use of constructive fantasy, you can eventually become adept at:

- relaxation via imagery
- avoidance of unconstructive/destructive food fantasizing
- success in controlling eating behaviors

Frustrated? Try Fantasy F:

Imagine yourself at the seashore, the waves lapping gently at the shoreline. Seagulls float overhead, and the sun is gently sinking toward the ocean. It is still and peaceful, and you are relaxed. A slight breeze gently ruffles your hair. You smile, and you are at peace. You are calm and serene.

Nervous? Try Fantasy N:

Imagine yourself floating on a soft mound of shaving cream. It is cool and soothing, and you let yourself sink in. Each muscle is relaxed, your eyes are closed, and you smile. Your heartbeat is gentle, you are still, and totally relaxed.

Depressed? Try Fantasy D:

Imagine yourself in a warm, pleasant room surrounded by your favorite people—friends, relatives, idols. It is a special party which is being given for you, because you are loved. You are smiling, everyone is happy and relaxed. You feel radiant.

Tempted by some delectable foodstuff?
Try Fantasy T:

Imagine yourself stepping onto a scale, and the dial turns directly to your desired weight...and stops. You smile, and reflect on the struggle of dieting and your own determination. You are proud of yourself, and feel warm all over.

Are you feeling angry, stressed, bored, fatigued, tempted by eating cues all around you? Relax for a minute or two, and flash onto your own inner television screen a constructive fantasy that you create yourself. Do you find yourself fantasizing about food? Again, try to relax and concentrate instead on constructive imagery. Fantasy can be used for fun, and to fight fat as well!

STEP 6: HOME MENU PLANNING

Meal planning is an essential component of your Nutri-Plan diet plan POA. By planning out your food intake, you can better control your eating behaviors by minimizing:

- impulse eating
- haphazard menu patterns
- excessive caloric intake
- inappropriate intakes of allowed daily food group servings

Use the meal pattern and serving sizes given in your Nutri-Plan diet plan (Day Sixteen) to assist you in planning ahead the foods and amounts you want to include on Day Eighteen. Record your menu plan in the chart that follows. The sample menu below illustrates the process for you.

In the Comments column, record any planned deviations from your meal pattern. You can switch food group servings between meals (eg, if you have an extra grain at lunch, simply delete one grain serving at supper), but to ensure a well-balanced diet, you should avoid switching one food group for another (eg, 1 grain + 1 fruit is not interchangeable with 2 meats). How do you think your POA worked out?

Day Eighteen Sample Menu Plan
(1200 Calorie Nutri-Plan Diet Plan)

Meal Pattern (see Day Sixteen)	Menu	Comments
Breakfast		
1 Grain	oatmeal, ½ cup	
½ cup Milk	skim milk, ½ cup	
1 Fruit	orange juice, ½ cup	
Lunch		
1 Meat	sandwich: 1 frankfurter	
1 Fat	with mustard	
2 Grain	on a bun	
1 Milk	yogurt, low-fat, 1 cup	extra ½ Fat
1 Fruit	with strawberries, 1 cup	
Supper		
4 Meat	4 oz broiled chicken	
2 Veg	1 cup broccoli with	
2 Fat	1 tsp margarine*	*only 1½ Fats (to make
1 Grain	sm baked potato with	up for the extra ½ Fat
	1 tbsp sour cream*	at lunch)
1 Fruit	½ cup pineapple with	
Luxury	angel food cake, sm piece	
Snacks		
1 Fruit	banana shake: ½ banana	
½ Milk	½ cup skim milk	
	crushed ice	
1 Grain	3 cups popcorn	

STEP 7: DAY EIGHTEEN PLAN

Follow your Day Eighteen menu plan. Be sure to record any planned deviations from your menu pattern in the Comments column. At the end of Day Eighteen, use red ink to circle any planned foods which were not included, and write in any unplanned foods you may have eaten. How closely were you able to approximate your menu plan? Why were the foods you circled omitted? Why did you eat the unplanned items? Quite often, changes in menu plans are unavoidable; try to make wise food selections when substitution for planned menu items is necessary. When allowed daily food group servings are omitted, try to include them at a later meal or snack. Be careful to count your fat servings properly.

At the end of Day Eighteen, devise a menu plan for Day Nineteen. Use the meal pattern and serving sizes given in your Nutri-Plan diet plan (Day Sixteen) to assist you. Follow the guidelines given in Step 6. How closely can you approximate your menu plan for Day Nineteen? What were the reasons for any unplanned deviations? The number of items circled in red ink will serve to illustrate the extent of your success in menu adherence on Day Nineteen. Remember, the better you are at making the POA at home, and the more diligent you are in devising and adhering to your menu plan, the closer you will come to obtaining the well-balanced diet designed to suit your personal needs.

Day Eighteen Menu Plan
(_____ Calorie Nutri-Plan Diet Plan)

Meal Pattern (See Day Sixteen)	Menu	Comments
Breakfast		
Lunch		
Supper		
Snacks		

Day Nineteen Menu Planner
(_____ Calorie Nutri-Plan Diet Plan)

Meal Pattern (see Day Sixteen)	Menu	Comments
Breakfast		
Lunch		
Supper		
Snacks		

Note: More information and guidelines concerning menu planning are given on Day Twenty-Two.

DAY NINETEEN

NUTRITION—IN THE SUPERMARKET

STEP 1: TO MARKET, TO MARKET

Once you have devised your menu plan, the next step is to purchase the foods and beverages required to meet your needs. With over 10,000 different items available in the typical supermarket from which you must choose, wise food selection may appear to be a difficult task.

When you shop for food, do you usually follow any of the basic guidelines listed below? Check (✓) to indicate how often, if ever, you:

the menu plans for Days Eighteen and Nineteen. Note, however, that Days Twenty through Twenty-Two are not to be included in your Nutri-Plan diet diary, but are to be planned out by you in the tri-out menu planner in this chapter.

Also, note that the tri-out menu planner for Days Twenty through Twenty-Two is designed slightly differently from the menu plan you utilized for Days Eighteen and Nineteen.

Often	Sometimes	Never	
☐	☐	☐	Plan menus in advance.
☐	☐	☐	Make a shopping list.
☐	☐	☐	Follow your shopping list without deviations, and avoid impulse purchases.
☐	☐	☐	Avoid familial persuasions and supermarket enticements.
☐	☐	☐	Purchase only low-calorie, high-nutrient snack foods.
☐	☐	☐	Purchase only required amounts to avoid leftovers.
☐	☐	☐	Avoid shopping when hungry.
☐	☐	☐	Read labels carefully to check for ingredients, serving size, nutrients, and calorie contents.
☐	☐	☐	Use extra care in checking labels on "dietetic" foods.
☐	☐	☐	Shop at consumer-oriented supermarkets.

STEP 2: TRI-OUT MENU PLANNER

Daily menu planning is a simple, practical method to ensure the intake of all of your nutrient needs. But daily food shopping would be unnecessarily time-consuming and expensive. Therefore, advanced planning of a few days of meals with accompanying food shopping lists proves more efficient, less costly, and ultimately less wasteful.

You can begin by devising in advance the menu plan for each of three days. Plan out your food and beverage intakes and the amounts for Day Twenty through Day Twenty-Two. It is not necessary to be overly specific and detailed, however. Simply use the same method you already utilized in devising

After each meal or snack eaten on Days Twenty through Twenty-Two, use red ink to circle any planned foods not eaten, and to write in any foods eaten which were not included in your tri-out menu planner. The number of items in red ink will serve to illustrate the extent of your success in menu adherence.

If you find that your actual intake is consistently and significantly different from your tri-out menu planner, you may eventually want to try one or more of the following alternatives:

- Plan only one or two days at a time.
- Devise a more general menu plan (with less specifics for you to vary from).

- Alter your meal pattern to better suit your intake habits.
- Adjust your calorie level to lessen the degree of deviation.

Be careful, however, that any alterations you make—in your tri-out menu planner, meal pattern, or Nutri-Plan diet plan—will be beneficial, not detrimental to your personal diet goals. Make your menu goals realistic. Avoid trying to do too much all at once: repeated failure can lead to diet depression and the desire to simply return to old eating patterns. On the other hand, avoid allowing yourself too much leeway: excessive flexibility can lead to undesirable diet deviations and may ultimately result in overall failure to improve your diet.

Try to create menus which differ from day to day, and to include in each day a variety of different foodstuffs. Remember that a well-balanced diet is a varied diet which includes moderate amounts of many different foods. And in planning your menus, be sure to consider the seasons and the types of foods available to you. For example, if

strawberries are in season, you may want to include them in several meals or snacks in a variety of forms (on hot cereal, in low-fat yogurt, etc).

Two sample tri-out menu planners have been completed below, to further illustrate the three-day menu planning process. Explanatory notes are given for each day's menu.

STEP 3: LIST MAKING

By referring to your tri-out menu planner, you can devise a well-organized shopping list that will simplify food selection in the supermarket. By adhering to your shopping list, you may be able to:

- avoid impulse purchases
- deal effectively with familial requests for specific purchases
- reduce or eliminate the high-calorie, low-nutrient foodstuffs available in your home.

Two Sample Tri-Out Menu Planners
(1000 Calorie Nutri-Plan Diet Plan)

Sample One

Meal	Day Twenty	Day Twenty-One	Day Twenty-Two
BREAKFAST	½ cup oatmeal with 2 tbsp raisins and ½ cup skim milk coffee, black	¾ cup shredded wheat with ¾ cup fresh strawberries and ½ cup skim milk coffee, black	1 sl whole wheat toast 10 to 12 cherries in ½ cup low-fat yogurt coffee, black
LUNCH	Open face sandwich: ½ whole wheat bagel ¼ cup tuna 2 tsp low-calorie mayo 1 cup skim milk orange	Open face sandwich: mini whole wheat pita 1 oz chicken, chopped 2 tsp low-calorie mayo lettuce 1 cup skim milk ½ sm banana	Chef's salad: 1 oz Swiss cheese 1 oz sl turkey lettuce bed lemon and vinegar 3 whole wheat melba toasts club soda
SUPPER	3 oz chicken wings, broiled with lemon and spices salad: lettuce ½ cup mixed raw vegetables lemon and vinegar ½ cup broccoli sm baked potato with 1 tbsp sour cream	3½ oz dry wine 3 oz roast turkey salad: lettuce ½ cup mixed raw vegetables 1 tbsp French dressing ½ cup asparagus 1 sm sweet potato 1 tsp margarine	Stuffed zucchini: 3 oz lean beef ¾ oz part-skim mozzarella ½ cup brown rice 3 crushed wheat melba toasts salad: lettuce ½ cup mixed vegetables ½ cup ice cream
SNACKS	3 cups popcorn with ½ oz parmesan cheese club soda	½ cup skim milk 3 arrowroots	orange

Explanatory Notes

Day	Breakfast	Lunch	Supper	Snacks
Twenty			½ Fat in sour cream + 1 Fat in ice cream +	½ Fat in parmesan cheese
Twenty-One				
Twenty-Two	½ Fat in yogurt +		½ Fat in part-skim mozzarella cheese +	1 Fat in ice cream
Twenty-Three	½ Fat in part-skim mozzarella cheese +	No Grain	½ Fat in dressing 2 Grain in 1 cup spaghetti	
Twenty-Four		1 Fat in mayonnaise + 1 Fat in yogurt + No Grain 1 Veg in celery, pepper + No Milk	1 Fat in part-skim mozzarella cheese 2 Grain in 2 sl pizza 1 Veg in salad 1 Milk in cheese	
Twenty-Five			½ Fat in dressing +	½ Fat in parmesan cheese

Sample Two

Meal	Day Twenty-Three	Day Twenty-Four	Day Twenty-Five
BREAKFAST	1 sl whole wheat toast with ¾ oz cheese, part-skim, melted ½ grapefruit coffee, black	½ cup oatmeal with ½ sm banana, sliced and ½ cup skim milk coffee, black	¾ cup shredded wheat with ½ cup skim milk ½ grapefruit coffee, black
LUNCH	Egg salad sandwich: ½ whole wheat bagel 1 egg, hard boiled 2 tsp low-calorie mayo lettuce 1 cup skim milk	Tuna salad: ¼ cup tuna 2 tsp low-calorie mayo ½ cup chopped celery, pepper lettuce bed fresh peach club soda	Open face sandwich: mini whole wheat pita ¼ cup low-fat cottage cheese 1 oz cheddar cheese, melted lettuce orange slices
SUPPER	3½ oz dry wine 1 cup whole wheat spaghetti with 3 oz shrimp in ½ cup tomato sauce salad: lettuce ½ cup mixed raw vegetables 1 tbsp blue cheese dressing	Pizza,* whole wheat, 2 sl (with 1½ oz part-skim cheese) 12 oz "light" beer salad: lettuce ½ cup mixed raw vegetables lemon and vinegar	3½ oz dry wine 3 oz cod, broiled salad: lettuce ½ cup mixed raw vegetables low-calorie dressing ½ cup broccoli 1 sm baked potato 1 tsp margarine
SNACKS	Thin Shake—blend: ½ cup skim milk ¾ cup strawberries crushed ice	½ cup skim milk 3 arrowroots	3 cups popcorn with ½ oz parmesan cheese club soda

*For pizza recipe, see Day Twenty-One.

Your Tri-Out Menu Planner
(_____ Calorie Nutri-Plan Diet Plan)

Meal	Day Twenty	Day Twenty-One	Day Twenty-Two
B R E A K F A S T			
L U N C H			
S U P P E R			
S N A C K S			

You may want to use the shopping list outliner given in this chapter to assist you in organizing a shopping list which is coordinated with your tri-out menu planner for Days Twenty through Twenty-Two. Foods included on your tri-out menu planner that you may already have on hand need not be added to your shopping list. Remember to add in required seasonings, paper goods, cleaning products, foods for family members, and other items usually purchased in the supermarket but not included in your tri-out menu planner. Proper menu planning utilizing organized shopping lists can be the key to both diet success and supermarket savings.

A sample shopping list outliner has been completed for you, using the two sample tri-out menu planners, to further illustrate the preparation of organized shopping lists. Compare the foods on the sample list to those included in the sample planner to determine:

- What foods are missing from the list? _____

_____

- What extra items are included on the list? _____

_____

After studying the sample shopping list outliner, complete your own list by referring to your tri-out menu planner for Days Twenty through Twenty-Two. Did you leave out any foods from your planner? Was this intentional (you had the items on hand) or accidental? Did you add any extra items to your list? Was this intentional (seasonings, paper goods, cleaning products, foods for family members, etc) or accidental?

Sample Shopping List Outliner
For Sample Tri-Out Menu Planner

Food	Amount
Fruit	
oranges	3
raisins	small box
strawberries, fresh	pint box
cherries, fresh	pint box
grapefruit	1
banana	1
peach, fresh	1
lemon	1
Vegetables	
broccoli	1 head
lettuce	2 to 3 heads
tomatoes*	2 to 3
zucchini	1 med
asparagus	small bunch
celery*	1 bunch
mushrooms	pint box
green pepper*	2 to 3
onions*	6 small
tomato sauce	small jar

Sample Shoppng List Outliner *(Continued)*

Food	Amount
Grains	
whole wheat bread	1 loaf
whole wheat pitas, mini	2 rounds
oats, rolled	small box
shredded wheat cereal	small box
whole wheat bagel	1
arrowroots	small box
brown rice	small box
potatoes	2 small
sweet potato	1 small
spaghetti, whole wheat	small box
whole wheat melba toasts	small box
popcorn	small bag
whole wheat flour	1 pound
Milk and Cheese	
skim milk	½ gallon
yogurt, low-fat	1 cup
cheese, part-skim mozzarella	3 oz
cheese, cheddar	1 oz
cheese, Swiss	1 oz
parmesan cheese, grated	small jar
Meat	
chicken wings	¼ lb
turkey, roaster	¼ lb
beef, lean	¼ lb
shrimp	3 oz
tuna, in water	7 oz can
cod	¼ lb
Alternates	
low-fat cottage cheese	½ pint
eggs	½ doz
Fats	
salad dressing, French	1 bottle
salad dressing, Italian	1 bottle
salad dressing, low-calorie	1 bottle
margarine	1 tub
low-calorie mayonnaise	1 jar
sour cream	½ pint
Beverages	
coffee, instant	small jar
wine, dry	1 quart
beer, "light"	6-pack
club soda	2 quarts
diet soft drink	1 quart
Luxury	
ice cream	½ pint
angel food cake	1 small
Miscellaneous	
aluminum foil	
napkins	
curry powder	
oregano	
garlic powder	
baby food	

Note: List calculated to serve one.
*for mixed vegetables

Note: Missing—coffee, vinegar (had on hand)
Extra—aluminum foil, paper napkins, seasonings, baby food, diet soft drink (items not on Planner)

Shopping List Outliner
For Tri-out Menu Planner
Days Twenty through Twenty-Two

Food	Amount
Fruit	
Vegetables	
Grains	
Milk and Cheese	

Shopping List Outliner *(Continued)*

Food	Amount
Meat	
Alternates	
Fats	
Beverages	
Luxury	
Miscellaneous	

STEP 4: MAPPING YOUR MARKET

A shopping list is ineffective unless it is used properly. Use your food shopping list as both a guide to wise food selection and a reminder of your particular diet goals. And try not to let environmental influences affect your shopping behaviors. Be wary of the possible detrimental effects of:

- advertising
- familial food requests
- tempting food displays and other types of supermarket psychology

Just remember that you are in control of your food selections and purchases. Use the supermarket psychology map illustrated below in order to identify possible supermarket pitfalls, and to identify ways you might save food dollars.

STEP 5: ARE YOU ABLE TO READ A FOOD LABEL?

All food labels must provide certain facts:

- product name
- name and address of manufacturer, packer, or distributor
- net weight or net contents

SUPERMARKET PSYCHOLOGY MAP

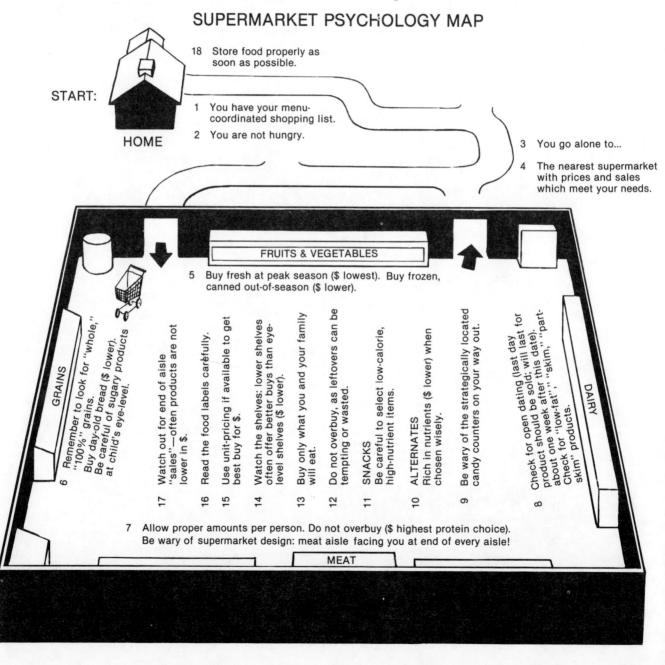

START:

HOME

18 Store food properly as soon as possible.

1 You have your menu-coordinated shopping list.

2 You are not hungry.

3 You go alone to...

4 The nearest supermarket with prices and sales which meet your needs.

FRUITS & VEGETABLES

5 Buy fresh at peak season ($ lowest). Buy frozen, canned out-of-season ($ lower).

GRAINS

6 Remember to look for "whole," "100%" grains. Buy day-old bread ($ lower). Be careful of sugary products at child's eye-level.

17 Watch out for end of aisle "sales"—often products are not lower in $.

16 Read the food labels carefully.

15 Use unit-pricing if available to get best buy for $.

14 Watch the shelves: lower shelves often offer better buys than eye-level shelves ($ lower).

13 Buy only what you and your family will eat.

12 Do not overbuy, as leftovers can be tempting or wasted.

11 SNACKS Be careful to select low-calorie, high-nutrient items.

10 ALTERNATES Rich in nutrients ($ lower) when chosen wisely.

9 Be wary of the strategically located candy counters on your way out.

8 Check for open dating (last day product should be sold; will last for about one week after this date). Check for "low-fat", "skim", "part-skim" products.

DAIRY

7 Allow proper amounts per person. Do not overbuy ($ highest protein choice). Be wary of supermarket design: meat aisle facing you at end of every aisle!

MEAT

Most food labels also include a list of ingredients:

- listed in order of amounts present in the product —the predominant ingredient is listed first, the ingredient present in the second largest amount listed next, and so on down the list as ingredient quantities lessen.
- with additives listed—but particular colors and flavors do not have to be identified (only "artificial color" or "artificial flavor" need be listed).

Certain foods have been given a "Standard of Identity" by the US Food and Drug Administration and must contain certain mandatory ingredients. Manufacturers can, and do, add other ingredients as well; we have no way of knowing exactly what these products contain, unless we write to the manufacturer.

US government regulations require that the labels of all foods with added nutrients, and any food for which a nutrition claim is made, must include nutrition information. Food processors may also choose to voluntarily provide nutrition information on foods which do not require nutrition labeling.

Nutrition labels provide product information including the number of:

- calories per serving
- grams of protein per serving
- grams of carbohydrate per serving
- grams of fat per serving
- servings (with serving sizes)

Nutrition labels also list the percentage of the US Recommended Daily Allowances for protein, and for seven essential vitamins and minerals. Some manufacturers also list other vitamins and/or minerals present, and it has recently become popular to also provide information on the sodium, cholesterol, and/or fatty acid (polyunsaturated vs saturated fats) contents.

Certain foods are graded by the US Department of Agriculture. Grading is based on the following criteria:

- taste
- appearance
- texture

The grades, present in the form of standardized symbols, do not reflect the nutritional quality of the product.

Certain other symbols you may notice on some food labels identify the four kinds of open dating, used to provide consumers with the opportunity to purchase only the freshest products:

- Freshness date—used on bakery products sold

at reduced cost to indicate that the item is not fresh but still edible.
- Expiration date—used for baby formulas and yeast to notify consumers of last date product should be used.
- Pack date—tells age of product by giving date of processing or packaging.
- Pull/Sell date—used on cold cuts, ice cream, milk, and yogurt to identify the last date the product should be sold; allows time for home storage.

Food labels may include several other symbols, including the following:

- Universal Product Code—appears as a band of vertical lines and allows automated check-out equipment to ring up sales and maintain inventory.
- Recall Code—provides information as to where and when products with especially long shelf lives were packaged; used in case of recall.
- "R"—indicates that the US Patent Office has registered the trademark used on the product.
- "C"—indicates that the US Copyright Office protects the label from reproduction without permission.
- "U"—indicates that use of the product is authorized by the Union of Orthodox Jewish Congregations of America.
- "K"—indicates that the product is Kosher and complies with Jewish law.

Examine food labels available on foods present in your home. Are you able to locate on the food label the information discussed above and illustrated by the sample given on page 144?

STEP 6: WE NEED MORE ABLE FOOD LABELS

The terms used on food labels to describe the product are often confusing and/or misleading. Give your definitions for the following:

- "natural"
- "organic"
- "health food"
- "no preservatives"
- "sugar-free"
- "sugarless"
- "no added salt"
- "low-sodium"
- "low-cholesterol"
- "low-calorie"
- "reduced calorie"
- "dietetic"

144

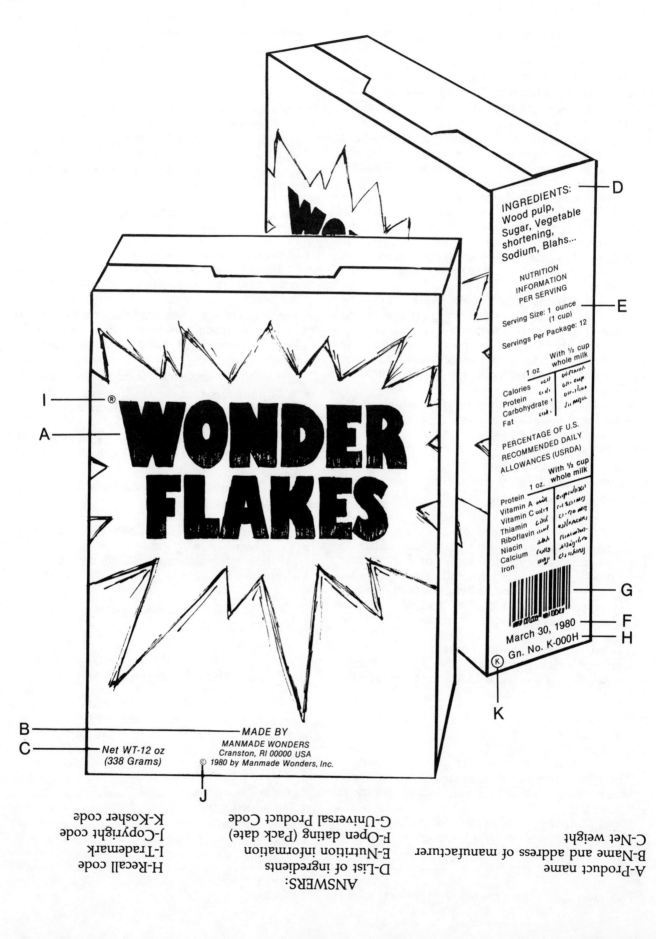

INGREDIENTS:
Wood pulp,
Sugar, Vegetable
shortening,
Sodium, Blahs...

D

NUTRITION
INFORMATION
PER SERVING

Serving Size: 1 ounce
(1 cup)

Servings Per Package: 12

E

	1 oz	With ½ cup whole milk
Calories		
Protein		
Carbohydrate		
Fat		

PERCENTAGE OF U.S.
RECOMMENDED DAILY
ALLOWANCES (USRDA)

	1 oz.	With ½ cup whole milk
Protein		
Vitamin A		
Vitamin C		
Thiamin		
Riboflavin		
Niacin		
Calcium		
Iron		

G

F

March 30, 1980

H

Gn. No. K-000H

K

WONDER FLAKES

I

A

B

C — Net WT-12 oz
(338 Grams)

MADE BY
MANMADE WONDERS
Cranston, RI 00000 USA
© 1980 by Manmade Wonders, Inc.

J

ANSWERS:

A-Product name
B-Name and address of manufacturer
C-Net weight

D-List of ingredients
E-Nutrition information
F-Open dating (Pack date)
G-Universal Product Code

H-Recall code
I-Trademark
J-Copyright code
K-Kosher code

The US Food and Drug Administration has issued rulings on the definitions for certain terms commonly used on food labels. At the present time, however, the laws are loose and we still can find products like potato chips labeled "natural" and high-calorie candy bars labeled as "dietetic."

The government is currently involved in the development of an overall food labeling policy which would assist consumers by lessening the amount of misleading product claims. Federal agencies and consumer groups are proposing that food labels be required to contain:

- a statement to explain that ingredients are listed in order of predominance
- information on sodium and sugar contents
- defined terms for low/reduced cholesterol and low/reduced sodium
- ingredient listings for standardized foods
- identification of specific spices, colors, and flavors by name
- specific sources of fat (on foods with fat contents over 10%)
- simpler nutrition labeling

It is only a matter of time before food labels will be easier to interpret. Until then, however, we need to read food labels carefully, in order to assess validity, identify any missing information, and determine all possible uses. The following definitions may assist you in the label interpretation process:

- "Natural"—most anything can be so labeled and thereby appeal to our health-conscious public; new labels may restrict use of this term to minimally processed products free of artificial ingredients and chemical additives.
- "Organic"—a substance can be so defined if it contains carbon, which all living substances (including plants and animals) contain; new law may require that use of this term be restricted to foods grown without use of synthetic fertilizers or pesticides.
- "Health food"—any food can support health, yet no food directly supplies health; use of this term should be eliminated, as it supports nutrition myths and high food costs.
- "No preservatives"—this label often adorns many foods which do not normally require preservatives, such as canned or heat-treated products; used to imply safety, the product may actually have a decreased shelf life and should be checked carefully as to freshness.
- "Sugar-free" or "sugarless"—these products do not contain table sugar, but may contain any of the following other sugars: glucose, fructose, maltose, mannose, ribose, lactose, hexitol, mannitol, xylitol, sorbitol; contrary to popular belief, these sugars provide as many calories per serving as table sugar.
- "No added salt"—the product may be naturally high in sodium or prepared with sodium-rich compounds.
- "Low sodium/low cholesterol"—standards are to be set which will define "low"; eventually, products may list the mg/serving.
- "Low calorie/reduced calorie"—recent law requires that products labeled as "low calorie" must contain no more than 40 calories per serving, and those labeled as "reduced calorie" must contain one third fewer calories than their non-diet counterparts.
- "Dietetic"—since there exists no consistent meaning for this term, products so labeled may contain an altered caloric content, less sodium, a decreased amount of cholesterol, or may simply lack added table sugar; until this term is banned or legally defined, extra care should be taken in interpreting "dietetic" labels.

STEP 7: WHERE TO MARKET, TO MARKET

Due to misleading food claims, inflation, and the multitude of non-nutritious foods available, should we avoid supermarkets in favor of specialty shops and health food stores?   ☐ Yes   ☐ No

Your local supermarket is actually not the enemy of a well-balanced diet. And although most supermarkets have room for improvement, wise food selections can be made at relatively low costs to provide the educated shopper with a nutritionally balanced diet. If you shop wisely for wholesome foods, there is no need to pay the high prices charged by specialty shops and health food stores. In fact, several supermarket chains now employ nutritionists, home economists, and consumer specialists to assist shoppers in their decision making. Some examples of on-going, in-store nutrition education programs include:

- Consumers Cooperative of Berkeley, Inc—Staff home economists educate shoppers using in-store signs and a free weekly newsletter. Many special consumer requests have been met by accommodating employees, including the removal of candy from check-out areas, and the availability of specialty nutrition items such as bulk grains.
- Giant Foods, Inc (Washington, DC/Baltimore area)—A program entitled "Foods for Health" was developed in conjunction with the National Heart, Lung, and Blood Institute. "Foods for Health" emphasizes heart health and offers a weekly nutrition newsletter. Changes in food selection are being monitored, and results may be used to demonstrate the value of in-store nutrition education programs.

• Purity Supreme Supermarkets, Inc—This New England supermarket chain offers "Food for Fitness," a nutrition education program intended for both consumers and health professionals. "Food for Fitness" identifies, through shelf labels and brochures, those products which fit into four categories: no added sugar, no added salt, calorie controlled, and fat modified. "Food for Fitness" can assist nutrition-conscious shoppers, as well as those with special dietary needs. The program has been made available (at no cost) to area health professionals for assistance in diet counseling.

Check the supermarkets in your area. You may be pleasantly surprised to find that they offer nutrition information, consumer assistance, and a variety of nutritious foods at affordable prices.

Are any nutrition information materials offered at the supermarket where you normally shop? If so, what exactly is available?

STEP 8: DAY NINETEEN PLAN

Using your tri-out menu planner and your correlated shopping list, shop at your local supermarket for those products required on Days Twenty through Twenty-Two. Did you buy every item on your list? Did you purchase any unplanned items? From the list below, identify (✓) those wise food shopping guidelines which you were able to employ. After all, the wise shopper is a healthy, thrifty, happy shopper!

Yes No

☐ ☐ I planned three days of menus in advance, using the tri-out menu planner.

☐ ☐ Using the planner and the shopping list outliner, I devised an organized shopping list.

☐ ☐ I followed the list and made no deviations or impulse purchases.

☐ ☐ I avoided familial persuasions by shopping alone (or with sheer determination).

☐ ☐ I was careful to avoid supermarket temptations.

☐ ☐ I bought only the required amounts of foodstuffs.

☐ ☐ I was not hungry when I shopped.

☐ ☐ I read labels carefully to check for ingredients, serving sizes, nutrient and caloric contents. I also checked for open dating, fresh quality, and the best prices.

☐ ☐ I avoided or used extra care in the selection of "dietetic" foods.

☐ ☐ I discovered that my supermarket has a consumer department offering nutrition education services.

Remember to follow your menu planner for Day Nineteen. At the end of Day Nineteen, examine any deviations you made from your planner. How closely did you approximate your menu plan for Day Nineteen? What were the reasons for any unplanned deviations? Could poor shopping habits prior to Day Nineteen have contributed to inappropriate food selections (eg, not enough nutritious foods on hand, high-calorie snack items readily available)?

DAY TWENTY

NUTRITION—AND DINING OUT

STEP 1: DIET VS DINING OUT

Special dining situations—such as restaurant dining, eating at work, and social dining—present a host of new eating problems. Restaurants offer many different tempting foods in large quantities and in an atmosphere conducive to relaxed, unlimited eating. When at work, you can delay tasks and socialize with co-workers in eating situations. And in social situations, you are usually expected, if not almost forced, to over-indulge. Holidays, vacations, and travel experiences are exceptionally conducive to the intake of excessive quantities of food, many of which fit into the high-calorie, low-nutrient category.

The main dietary difficulty with dining out is not just that food is the main focus, but that we overemphasize the importance of food and ignore the value in using food wisely.

There are two simple rules to follow when dining out, whether at a restaurant, at work, or as a house or party guest:

1) Plan ahead.
2) Be moderate.

By following these two rules, your dining out experiences are more apt to be enjoyable social events, and less apt to turn into overindulgent food orgies.

Consider your own eating behaviors when dining out, and answer True or False to the following statements:

True	False	
☐	☐	I tend to overeat in restaurants because I try to get my money's worth.
☐	☐	I tend to choose rich menu items which I would never eat at home.
☐	☐	I often visit "eat-all-you-want" restaurants in order to receive unlimited helpings.
☐	☐	I often visit restaurants that specialize in fried foods (fried meats, fish, poultry, vegetables, or donuts).
☐	☐	I go to fast food restaurants at least once a month.
☐	☐	I tend to indulge in high-calorie coffee breaks at work.

True	False	
☐	☐	I often have high-calorie meals during work (especially when on an expense account).
☐	☐	In a social situation, I tend to consume more alcoholic beverages than usual.
☐	☐	As a guest, I always eat what is served to avoid being rude.
☐	☐	I usually feel insulted or rejected when a guest refuses food or drink.
☐	☐	I always "blow"/go off my diet on holidays.
☐	☐	I always "blow"/go off my diet on vacations or when traveling.

STEP 2: RESTAURANT RULES

Eating is only one component of the social event of restaurant dining. Restaurants can also offer:

- a relaxed atmosphere
- time away from home
- the opportunity to avoid cooking and clean-up
- a chance to socialize

Thus, when dining out, you pay for more than the food. You can get your money's worth by enjoying yourself without overindulging. You may want to use some of the following suggestions whenever you dine in a restaurant:

Plan Ahead

- Choose restaurants that offer nutritious foods in moderate portions. Avoid restaurants conducive to overindulging (such as those with eat-all-you-want specials) and places with menus limited to high-calorie, low-nutrient fast foods (such as fried clam stands).
- Before you go to a restaurant, decide on your general order (eg, broiled fish or chicken) and what you will avoid (eg, fried foods and sauces).
- For an upcoming special meal, budget nutrients and calories; you may want to plan out a menu pattern in which some of your allowed daily

food group servings are saved for the special meal (this means adjusting for that particular day, not skimping for weeks!).

• Do not dine out when ravenous because *everything* appears invitingly delicious; instead, have a small salad or some fruit before you go.

Be Moderate

• Select nutritious appetizers such as fresh fruits and vegetables and eat sparingly. Avoid fatty, salty, high-calorie choices such as chips, dips, and fried mushrooms.

• Try creating a meal around nutritious appetizers; simply add bread, salad, and a beverage.

• If you do not think that you can avoid overindulgence in bread and butter, keep it out of your reach, or ask the waiter to remove it from the table.

• Request that undesirable items not be served (eg, ask the waiter to hold the garlic toast, french fries, etc).

• Do not hesitate to ask for substitutions (eg, lettuce and tomato instead of potato chips). After all, you are the customer.

• Request that salad dressing be served on the side, so that you control the serving amounts; you may even want to bring along your own low-calorie brand.

• Avoid overindulging in alcoholic beverages. Have dry wine or "light" beer, or order fruit juice, club soda, even mineral water with a twist.

• Share your order with others, and/or bring home extras in a "doggie bag."

• Eat moderate amounts, and enjoy each dining out experience for what it is really worth.

STEP 3: RESTAURANT MENU SELECTION

The chart below and on the next pages summarizes the dos and don'ts for selecting foods from a restaurant menu, and may assist you to choose foods wisely when dining out.

Also, watch out for these high-calorie terms:
• buttered, butter sauce, buttery
• creamed, cream sauce, creamy
• au gratin, escalloped, in cheese sauce, parmigiana
• casserole, in gravy, pot pie, stew
• Bernaise, hollandaise, in white sauce
• crispy, deep fried, French fried, sauteed

Note that certain Dos may contain appreciable amounts of fat, sugar, salt, alcohol, and/or calories, but are acceptable on occasion in moderate amounts. Use your nutrition know-how and some practical sense in making dining out decisions. The choice, as always, is yours.

STEP 4: A WORK-ING DIET PLAN

For many people, the office is a high-calorie trap, with coffee breaks, the building cafeteria, local restaurants, and countless office social events which can contribute to an unbalanced dietary intake. If you are encountering on-the-job eating problems, you may want to try some of the following suggestions:

Plan Ahead

• Eat a well-balanced diet at home. A full stomach can make it easier to resist Danish and donuts later on.

• Do not keep food at your desk, and try to avoid forming the habit of eating at your desk— even at lunchtime. Find an alternate place to eat so that you will not associate working at your desk with nibbling on food.

• Avoid joining coffee clubs with co-workers if "goodies" are provided. After all, it is difficult to resist getting your money's worth.

• Plan activities for lunchtime and work breaks. Try to exercise during these time periods; even a brisk walk can use up calories and alleviate boredom (more about exercise on Day Twenty-Five).

		Dos	Don'ts
A W E S O M E	A P P E T I Z E R S	fresh fruits fresh juices fresh vegetables (crudités) seafood cocktail*	avocado butter crackers chips dips fried foods nuts patés processed cheeses (minimize intake of all cheeses)

• Use your imagination in planning non-food gifts for co-workers: flowers, a poem, or a homemade craft are often more appealing and always less caloric than a cake or box of candy. You may even interest co-workers in improving their own diets!

• Plan ahead for special dinners and office parties. If you have a general idea of the menu ahead of time, you can plan the day's meals accordingly. Remember to avoid these events when you are ravenous, lest you end up on an hors d'oeuvres orgy!

		Dos	Don'ts
S U B T L E	S O U P S	clear broth* clear consommé* gazpacho* vegetable broth*	bean soups cheese soups chowders cream soups French onion soup sweetened fruit soups
S L I N K Y	S A L A D S	Caesar's salad Chef's salad (lean meats and cheeses) seafood salad spinach salad (avoid bacon) tossed salad light/diet dressings* oil and vinegar	cole slaw (except vinegar-based) mayonnaise-based salads (including meat, egg, fish, potato, and Waldorf salads) bacon bits creamy dressings
B R E A K I N'	B R E A D	bagels breadsticks* crackers* English muffins French bread hard rolls* Italian bread matzoth* pita bread sandwich breads tortillas wafers* whole grain breads and rolls	biscuits butter rolls Chinese noodles (fried) croissants Danish donuts French toast garlic bread muffins pancakes waffles
F I S H Y	F A R E	any variety prepared without added fat (Note: shrimp is high in cholesterol)	baked stuffed broiled in butter fishsticks fried, batter fried
P R I Z E	P O U L T R Y	chicken, Cornish hen, turkey; prepared without skin or added fat	duck, goose batter dipped fried parmigiana pot pies stews stuffed
H E A R T Y	M E A T S	lean cuts, well-trimmed; baked, boiled, broiled, or roasted without added fat (Note: organ meats are high in cholesterol)	prime cuts, untrimmed breaded fried ground gravies luncheon meats parmigiana pot pies stews

Be Moderate

• At office parties, keep intake of alcoholic beverages moderate. Try a dry wine, or "light" beer. You may even choose to drink fresh juice, club soda, or mineral water with a twist, and save yourself the difficulties associated with a next-day-hangover.

• Avoid the party-fare table if it contains only chips, dips, and rich desserts. Instead, munch lightly on fresh vegetable sticks and whole grain crackers; if your office parties never offer these items, bring them yourself.

• During coffee breaks, lunchtime, work hours, and after hours, be moderate in your food intake. A well-balanced diet can be obtained away from as well as in the home.

		Dos	Don'ts
A P P E T I Z I N G	A L T E R N A T E S	cottage cheese (preferably low-fat) dried beans and peas, prepared without added fat egg, boiled or poached (Note: eggs are high in cholesterol)	egg, fried or scrambled peanut butter omelets quiches souffles
P O T A T O	P I C K I N G S	baked boiled	cheese-baked chips French fried fried, fried skins hash browns mashed potato salad scalloped
V A R I O U S	V E G E T A B L E S	all plain	creamed fried sauced seasoned
F R U I T Y	F A R E	all plain	candied in liqueurs sweetened with cream toppings
D E L I G H T F U L	D E S S E R T S	fresh fruit angel food cake cookies, plain fruit ices gelatin ice cream, plain sherbet sponge cake (Note: eat small portions as are high in sugar content)	rich sweets

		Dos	Don'ts
L I P Q U E N C H I N G	L I Q U I D S	club soda coffee, tea diet soft drinks fruit juices "light" beer milk, low-fat or skim mineral water (Note: coffee, tea, and some diet soft drinks are high in caffeine content)	fruit-flavored drinks, sweet- ened lemonade, limeade milkshakes soft drinks stout, ales sweet mixers, liqueurs table wine
E X T R A S		catsup* cocktail sauce* cottage cheese, low-fat herbs, spices horseradish* hot sauce* lemon juice, lemon, lime mustard* pickles, unsweetened* vinegar yogurt, low-fat, plain	bacon butter, margarine cream cream cheese non-dairy creamers olives relishes salt sour cream sweeteners (honey, sugar, syrups) tartar sauce yogurt, sweetened

*Contain considerable amounts of sodium.

STEP 5: PARTY ON!

As a guest, you may often feel pressured to eat and drink all that is offered—in excessive amounts— lest you appear rude. You may feel torn between the following:

- desire to please/not to offend the host or hostess
- strong temptations to overindulge yourself
- desire to choose foods wisely

Often you must make compromises in your food choices, and constantly remind yourself that consumption of food and drink is not the best way to express your love for and acceptance of your host or hostess.

You may want to use some of the following suggestions whenever you attend a social gathering:

Plan Ahead

- Find out the menu ahead of time whenever possible. You may want to enlist the understanding and support of your host or hostess.
- Prepare effective responses for insistent hosts and hostesses (eg, "This is delicious, but I'm totally full"; "I'm saving room for the next delicious course"; "Thanks so much, but I think I'd prefer a glass of mineral water instead of another glass of bourbon—but I will take a twist").
- Budget nutrients and calories for the upcoming event; you may want to plan out a menu pattern in which some of your allowed daily food group servings are saved for the social event (this means adjusting for that particular day, not skimping for weeks!).
- Everything will appear temptingly delicious if you are hungry. Have a small salad or some fruit before subjecting yourself to those long, hors d'oeuvres-laden cocktail hours.

Be Moderate

- A buffet-style meal allows for freedom in food selection and control over portion sizes, making it easy to be moderate… or to really overindulge.
- It is not necessary to eat all that is served. Keep in mind that gratitude can be expressed through means other than food intake. Make a special effort to praise your host or hostess on topics other than culinary expertise.
- Keep intake of alcoholic beverages moderate as well. Stick to dry wines, "light" beers, or non-alcoholic selections such as juice or mineral water. You may find yourself in better shape for the drive home.

Note: "Do unto others as you would have them do unto you." Do not force food and drink on your guests, and remember that a rejection of your foodstuffs is not a rejection of you. Make nutritious, low-calorie items available. After all, your guests may be as health conscious as you are! And preparation of creative, delicious, nutritious party-fare can be an exciting challenge. You may want to begin experimenting with new recipes, such as those included on Days Twenty-One and Twenty-Three.

STEP 6: HOLIDAY AND TRAVEL FARE

It is usually quite difficult to avoid overindulgence during holiday time and on vacations. We tend to spend too much money, attend too many social events, stay up too late, and eat and drink too much. The wise individual learns how to budget money, time, and food intake in all situations, including holiday fests and vacation travels. Meals and snacks need not be plain and unfestive in order to be nutritious. We just need to be more careful in our food selections and more moderate in our serving sizes.

You may want to use some of the following suggestions whenever holidays occur, vacation time arrives, or travel opportunities arise:

Plan Ahead

- Have low-calorie, nutrient-rich foods on hand for guests.
- Plan menus in advance, whether at home, at a social event, or on the road.
- Bring along nutritious foods in case travel fare is scarce, inedible, and/or lacking in nutritional value.
- When visiting others or entertaining guests, inform them of your diet and health goals. Who knows? They may join you in your quest for improved health through proper nutrition.

Be Moderate

- Avoid rich party-fare, constant fast food indulgences, and other high-calorie, low-nutrient food selections when dining out during your holiday or vacation seasons. A week of pastry, dips, and double cheeseburgers may undo a month of well-balanced meals.
- Take the opportunity to plan special enjoyable activities that will not lead to eating misbehavior. Visit a museum, enjoy a hike, go to an arts and crafts fair. Plan a party with a new focus; instead of a Christmas eve dinner, why not wait and have a New Year's eve Las Vegas party? And how about giving a Fourth of July run-a-thon?

STEP 7: DAY TWENTY PLAN

For Day Twenty, follow your tri-out menu planner from Day Nineteen. At the end of Day Twenty, use red ink to circle all planned foods which were not included and to write in any unplanned items you may have eaten. How closely did you approximate your tri-out menu planner for Day Twenty? What were the reasons for any unplanned deviations? Were any of your unplanned eating behaviors due to:

- dining out in restaurants?
- dining out during office hours?
- coffee break goodies?
- office social events?
- holiday doings?
- vacation?
- traveling?

If you did deviate from your tri-out menu planner due to any of the above reasons, did you still make the wisest food selections possible under the circumstances?

Try the following Nutri-Plan New Diner activity to see just how easy it is to make wise food selections from a typical dinner menu. First, outline your planned breakfast and lunch allowed daily food group servings (from Day Sixteen) on the following chart. Then select those dinner choices which would best balance out the day's intake and meet the requirements of your Nutri-Plan diet plan. Do not be afraid to make some alterations in the dinner menu as given (eg, removal of one slice of bread from a sandwich, salad dressing on-the-side, broccoli without the hollandaise). You can also moderate the given serving sizes—offer some to others, or bring extras home in a "doggie bag." Use the suggestions given in Step 3 (Dos and Don'ts) in order to make wise food selections from the menu (on pages 154–155) at the Nutri-Plan New Diner.

Now, examine the Nutri-Plan New Diner menu in order to select foods which satisfy your food desires and meet the allowed daily food group servings which you have allotted for your dinner meal. Circle possible selections and record your final choices on the chart on the following page. And enjoy your dinner at the Nutri-Plan New Diner!

Wise food selections are quite possible and can prove to be highly enjoyable when dining out. Remember that a well-balanced diet includes a variety of foods in moderate amounts. What better way to increase the variety of your food intake than to dine in a variety of settings?

Your Planned Breakfast and Lunch Menus
(Dinner at Nutri-Plan New Diner)
_____ Calorie Nutri-Plan Diet Plan

Meal Pattern (see Day Sixteen)	Menu	Comments*
Breakfast		
Lunch		

*You may want to omit certain allowed daily food group servings from your breakfast and lunch meals, and save them to include at dinner.

Your Planned Dinner Menu
From Nutri-Plan New Diner

Meal Pattern (see Day Sixteen)	Menu Choices From Nutri-Plan New Diner Menu	Comments*
Dinner (Supper):		

*Explain any deviations from your dinner meal pattern. Describe any menu modifications you would make (eg, removal of one slice of bread from a sandwich). Were you able to approximate your Nutri-Plan diet plan, despite the enjoyable repast you ate at the Nutri-Plan New Diner? If not, what led to the deviations?

Nutri-Plan New Diner

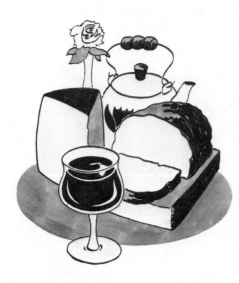

Awesome Appetizers

Carrot Juice Eye Opener
Grapefruit and Pineapple Juice Drink
Melon-filled Fresh Fruit Cup
Sherbety Fruit Cocktail

Jumbo Shrimp Cocktail
King Crab Leg
Oysters on the Half Shell

Escargots au Buerre
Avocado Dip 'n Taco Chips
Goose Paté on Butter Thins
Deep-Fried Mushrooms

Marinated Artichoke Hearts
White Asparagus Tips in Lemon Vinegar

Pastry Puffs: Cheese-filled, Salmon-filled,
              Creamed spinach-filled

Slinky Salads

Tossed Greens Salad
Nutri-Salad (includes skim milk cheeses,
  sliced chicken, assorted veggies, raisins, chickpeas)
Deep Sea Salad (includes fresh shrimp,
  crab, and lobster)
Waldorf Wonder (includes apples and walnuts)
Bleu Cheese Plate (assorted cheeses on
  bed of greens covered with thick bleu
  cheese dressing)
Hot German Potato Salad (a creamed dish with
  chunks of potato, egg, and bacon)
Popeye's Favorite (includes fresh spinach,
  mushrooms, and bacon bits)

All with choice of dressing: Creamy French,
Vinaigrette, Italian, Avocado, Bleu Cheese, Oil &
Vinegar.

Subtle Soups

Gruyère Onion Soup
Braised Vegetable Broth
Garden Gazpacho
Cream of Broccoli Soup
Chunky Fish Chowder
Beans n' Lentil Soup
Cold Cherry Soup

Breaking Bread

Homestyle Biscuits
Crusty French Bread
Garlic Bread
Bagels n' Cream Cheese
Homemade Muffins (Pecan, Corn, Berry)

Main Meals

Super Steak—10 oz of prime beef cooked to your desire
Veal Scallopini—thinly sliced, simmered with wine and mushrooms
King Crab Legs—large, succulent, fresh
Hearty Halibut—broiled in butter, baked stuffed, or batter fried
Jumbo Shrimp—broiled in butter, baked stuffed, or batter fried
Cape Scallops—broiled in butter, deep fried, or baked in a rich cheese sauce
Chicken Parmigiana—boneless breast of chicken which is batter dipped and layered with cheese
                   and tomato sauce
Chicken Marengo—tenderly broiled breast of chicken with homemade tomato sauce and garlic
Southern Fried Chicken—whole chicken fried in a crispy, spicy batter
Mama Mia's Lasagna—thick layers of cheese, noodles, and homemade tomato sauce
Spinach Soufflé—a puffed delicacy rich in eggs and creamed spinach
Dieter's De-Light—a 5 oz hamburger patty, served with cottage cheese and canned peaches
Today's Quiche—Swiss cheese 'n tomato, with ham chunks

Potato Pickings

Baked, with Sour Cream
French Fried Spuds
Heavenly Hash Browns
Cheese-stuffed Bakers
Escalloped Potato Plate

De-Lightful Desserts

Ice Cream or Sherbet (assorted flavors)
Angelfood Cake with Fudge Sauce
Fresh Strawberry Shortcake
Gelatin a la Whipped Creme
Ginger Snap Pudding

Various Vegetables

Asparagus au Gratin
Braised Celery Hearts
Honeyed Baby Carrots
Broccoli Hollandaise
French Fried Zucchini
Sautéed Mushrooms
Corn on the Cob (in season)

Fruity Fare

Poached Pears
Honey Baked Bananas
Assorted Fresh Fruit Tray
Fresh Berries n' Cream

Lip-Quenching Liquids

Assorted ales, beers, and wines (ask your waiter)
Lemonade   Milk
Cola   Coffee
Root Beer   Sanka
Ginger Ale   Tea
Diet Soft Drinks   Herbal Tea

Super-Saving-Sandwiches

All sandwiches are served on *your* choice of plain
or toasted white, wheat, rye, oatmeal or pita bread:

Cheddar 'n Bacon Burger   Tuna Fish Salad
Cheddar Burger   Chicken Salad
Naked Burger   Sliced Egg 'n Avocado
Grilled Cheese   Crabmeat Salad
Grilled Cheese 'n Tomato   Mixed Vegetable 'n Cheese
        Peanut Butter, Bacon, and Banana

◆

DAY TWENTY-ONE

SNACKING SMARTS

STEP 1: SNACK HABITS

Snacks can threaten dieting success if they are:

- Unplanned
- Low in nutritional value
- Eaten impulsively

Snacks are usually composed of tempting foods which heighten the urge to overeat. Most snacks are chosen from the Others Group and are high in:

- Fat
- Sugar
- Salt
- Alcohol

So, should we avoid snacks altogether? Should we limit ourselves to three meals, without any foodstuffs in between? In today's hurried world, filled with coffee breaks and cocktail hours, it would be difficult and burdensome to regiment ourselves to only three meals each day. Snacking, therefore, needs to be as healthful as it is practical.

Fortunately, snacks can contribute to the overall nutritional content of your diet. By selecting your snack foods as wisely as you do other foods you plan to consume, nutritious and delicious snacks can be built into the Nutri-Plan diet plan. In fact, snacks can become an integral component of your daily diet.

Examine the following statements, and select (✓) the answers that best apply to your snack habits:

Often True	Sometimes True	Never True	
☐	☐	☐	I do not buy high-calorie, low-nutrient snack foods.
☐	☐	☐	I do not go for long periods of time without eating (eg, 8 hours between lunch and dinner).
☐	☐	☐	I do not snack while engaged in other activities (eg, watching television, driving, talking on the phone, etc).
☐	☐	☐	I do not snack (or nibble) while preparing or cleaning up meals.
☐	☐	☐	I do not eat my snacks while standing up.
☐	☐	☐	I do not snack uncontrollably (ie, resulting in binges).
☐	☐	☐	I do not eat unplanned snacks.
☐	☐	☐	I include snacks as an integral component of my daily diet.

Unless you were able to select Often True for a majority of these statements, you may want to revise your snack habits.

STEP 2: YOUR SNACK HABITS

Snacks, like meals, can contribute valuable nutrients to your diet, and good health to your lifestyle. A moderate amount of nutrient-rich snack foods can serve as an important step in the path to a well-balanced diet.

In the chart below, list those snacks which you tend to eat most often. Indicate the number of calories per serving for each snack food (use a calorie chart from the references in Appendix C for assistance). Then consider each item carefully to determine why you enjoy it as a snack: taste? texture? ease of eating? convenience? habit? Indicate (✔) if these snack foods are high in nutritional value:

- Do not eat snacks when cued by your environment (eg, seeing a chocolate cake, smelling freshly baked cookies, etc).
- Eat snacks only when you are physically hungry.
- Eat your snacks while relaxed and sitting down (rather than standing by the refrigerator or while rushing about).
- Eat your snacks slowly—enjoy each mouthful.
- Bring nutritious snack foods from home for coffee breaks, movies, etc; you can thus avoid the urge to indulge in Danish, soft drinks, etc, and you may even improve your food budget as well.
- Make nutritious snacks an integral component of your daily diet.

Snack Foods	Calories per Serving	Nutrient Rich (✔)

To build snacks into your Nutri-Plan diet plan, follow the meal pattern given for your plan, and limit amounts to those indicated in the serving sizes (Day Sixteen). You may also want to try to revise any undesirable snack habits by incorporating the following suggestions into your own lifestyle:

- Avoid buying high-calorie, low-nutrient snack foods.
- Plan snacks carefully into your Nutri-Plan diet plan to avoid large gaps of time without food (over-hungry can lead to over-indulgence).
- Make snack-eating a sole activity, and avoid snacking while engaged in other activities (eg, watching television, driving, talking on the phone, etc).

STEP 3: YOUR SMART SNACKS

By planning snacks wisely, you can incorporate them into your Nutri-Plan diet plan and use "snack control" to avoid hunger pangs and end-of-the-day binges. You may choose to reduce your allowed daily food group servings at one or more meals, and substitute snacks. In fact, you may want to alter your meal pattern so that you are eating five or six small "meal-snacks" each day. And if you happen to miss out on some of your allowed daily food group servings, include them later on in the day as snacks.

Following are some snack suggestions—including recipes, approximate calories per serving, and daily food group serving equivalents. Note that caloric values are only estimates, and that daily food group serving equivalents are not always exactly equal to the caloric contents—any additional calories can be counted as extra or luxury calories. Why not make some of the following smart snacks (low in calories, high in nutritional value) part of your daily diet? You may find that you are healthier and happier because of it!

Fruited Yogurt—60 calories (1 Fruit)

3 sm bananas, sliced
¾ cup seedless grapes
½ cup blueberries
1 sm orange, peeled, in segments
1 cup low-fat yogurt
1 tsp vanilla
2 tsp honey
¼ cup orange juice, unsweetened

Combine fruit together in large bowl. Mix remaining ingredients together and stir into fruit. Toss lightly and refrigerate, covered, for an hour or more. Makes 10 (½ cup) servings.

Yogurt Crumble—125 calories (1 Fruit + ¼ Milk + ½ Fat)

½ cup low-fat yogurt
1 sm apple, grated
1 tbsp slivered almonds
1 tbsp raisins
2 graham cracker squares

Combine first four ingredients and mix well. Crumble grahams over top of yogurt mixture and serve. Serves 2.

Special Sundaes—140 calories (1 Fruit +1 Meat)

1 cup strawberries or
½ cup pineapple chunks, unsweetened
½ sm banana, split lengthwise
⅓ cup cottage cheese, uncreamed
1 tbsp defrosted, undiluted, frozen orange
  juice concentrate, unsweetened
1 tsp dried, unsweetened coconut
1 tsp wheat germ

Place fruit in shallow dish. Add scoop of cottage cheese. Top with juice. Sprinkle coconut and wheat germ over top. Serve chilled.

Bran 'n Date Quick Bread—85 calories (½ Grain + ½ Fat)

1½ cups whole wheat flour
1 tbsp baking powder
1 tsp salt
1½ cups unprocessed bran
½ cup chopped dates

1 egg
¾ cup skim milk
½ cup maple syrup
¼ cup vegetable oil

Mix dry ingredients together. Add remaining ingredients and mix together. Do not overbeat. Bake in an oiled loaf pan at 350° for 50 minutes or until done. Makes 24 slices.

Bran 'n Date Muffins—115 calories (1 Grain + 1 Fat)

¼ cup margarine
2 tbsp honey
⅔ cup skim milk
1 egg
¼ cup molasses
1 cup whole wheat flour
1 cup unprocessed bran
¼ cup wheat germ
1 tbsp baking powder
¼ tsp salt
12 dates, chopped

Beat first two ingredients together in large bowl. Blend in well milk, egg and molasses. Stir dry ingredients together and add to batter. Mix just until dry ingredients are moistened. Do not overbeat. Stir in dates. Fill paper-lined muffin tins ½ full. Bake at 400° for 15 minutes. Makes 15 muffins.

Blueberry Muffins—90 calories (1 Grain + ½ Fat)

2¼ cups whole wheat flour
¼ cup unprocessed bran
1¼ tsp baking soda
¼ tsp salt
1 egg
⅓ cup honey
¼ cup vegetable oil
1¾ cups buttermilk
1½ cups frozen blueberries, unsweetened

Mix together flour, bran, soda and salt. Beat together next four ingredients and stir into flour mixture, just enough to moisten. Do not overbeat. Fold blueberries into batter. Fill paper-lined muffin tins ½ full. Bake 20 minutes at 400°. Makes 24 small muffins.

Whole Wheat Muffins—110 calories (1 Grain + 1 Fat)

6 tbsp vegetable oil
¼ cup honey
1¼ cup skim milk
1 egg
1 cup whole wheat flour
¼ cup wheat germ

4 tsp baking powder
½ tsp salt

Preheat oven to 425°. Mix oil with honey. Add milk and egg and stir until well blended. In a large bowl, mix remaining ingredients together. Add liquid mixture, stirring quickly until mixed. Do not overbeat. Fill paper-lined muffin tins ⅔ full. Bake for 15 to 20 minutes or until done. Makes 15 muffins.

◆

Mock Guacamole—90 calories (1 Meat + ½ Fat)

¼ cup onion, chopped
1 tbsp vegetable oil
⅓ cup parsley, chopped
½ tsp basil
¼ tsp salt
⅛ tsp oregano
⅛ tsp cumin
1 sm clove garlic, crushed
¼ cup lemon juice
1 15-oz can garbanzo beans (chickpeas)
3 tbsp tahini (ground sesame seeds)

Drain beans and blend ¼ cup juice with other ingredients, except tahini, in blender until smooth. Add beans gradually, blending until smooth after each addition. Blend tahini into bean mixture. Chill. Makes 8 (¼ cup) servings. Serve with raw vegetables.

◆

Eggplant Dip—65 calories (1 Veg + 1 Fat)

¼ cup vegetable oil
1 lg eggplant, diced
2 med onions, diced
1 lg green pepper, diced
1 16-oz can tomatoes
½ tsp salt
⅛ tsp pepper
dash Worcestershire sauce
1 cup low-fat yogurt, plain
2 tbsp lemon juice
⅔ cup parsley, minced
½ 6-oz can tomato paste

Heat oil in a large skillet and sauté eggplant, onions, and pepper over medium heat, stirring occasionally until onions are translucent. Lower heat, add tomatoes, and cook until vegetables are tender. Cool to lukewarm. Stir remaining ingredients into vegetables and chill. Makes 16 (¼ cup) servings. Serve with whole wheat crackers or small wedges of whole wheat pita bread.

◆

Cucumber Dip—14 calories (1 Veg)

1 cucumber, peeled and seeded
1 cup low-fat yogurt
2 tsp lemon juice

1 clove garlic, minced
3 walnuts, minced
dash soy sauce
dash curry powder

Grate and drain cucumber well. Put in small bowl. Add remaining ingredients and mix well. Chill several hours before serving. Makes 16 (1 tbsp) servings. Serve with raw vegetables.

◆

Slim Shakes—125 calories (1 Fruit + 1 Milk)

1 cup skim milk
crushed ice cubes
2 tsp honey
1 cup strawberries or
½ cup blueberries or
2 dates, chopped or
½ sm banana, sliced

Beat ingredients together in blender until creamy and frothy. Serve at once. Makes one serving.

◆

Banana-Yogurt Sipper—150 calories (1 Fruit + ¾ Milk + ¾ Fat)

¾ cup low-fat yogurt, plain
½ sm banana, sliced
2 dates, chopped
¼ tsp vanilla

Mix in blender and chill. Serves one.

◆

Other Yogurt Sippers—150 calories (1 Fruit + ¾ Milk + ¾ Fat)

Substitute for banana and dates:
¼ cup orange juice and ¼ cup pineapple chunks
2 tbsp pineapple juice and ½ cup strawberries
1 cup blueberries and 2 ice cubes

◆

GORP—150 calories (2 Fruit + 2 Fat)

1¼ cups raisins
1 cup unsalted peanuts

Mix together. Store in baggies. Handy for trips.

◆

Celery Stuffers—75 calories (½ Fruit + 1 Veg + 1 Meat or 1 Fat)

2 lg stalks celery
4 tbsp low-fat cottage cheese or
1 tsp peanut butter
1 tbsp raisins

Spread celery with cottage cheese or peanut butter. Dot with raisins. Serves one.

◆

Whole Wheat Pizza-ettes—140 calories (1 Grain + ½ Milk + ¼ Fat)

1 whole wheat English muffin
2 tbsp tomato sauce
1½ oz part-skim mozzarella cheese
dash grated parmesan cheese

Spread 1 tbsp sauce on each muffin half. Top with mozzarella, sprinkle with parmesan, and broil 2 to 3 minutes until bubbly. Serves 2.

◆

Whole Wheat Pizza—150 calories (1 Grain + ½ Milk + ¾ Fat)

1 pkg dry yeast
1 cup warm water
2 cups whole wheat flour
1 cup all-purpose flour
½ tsp salt
2 tbsp vegetable oil
1 sm onion, minced
1 clove garlic, minced
1 tbsp vegetable oil
1 cup tomato sauce
1 tsp dried basil
1 tsp oregano
dash pepper
¼ lb part-skim mozzarella cheese, sliced
¼ cup grated parmesan cheese

Dissolve yeast in water for several minutes. Add next four ingredients to yeast and mix to make stiff dough. Cover, and let stand in warm place to rise. Brown onion and garlic in vegetable oil until golden. Add tomato sauce and seasonings and simmer 5 minutes. Divide dough, and place each half in 2 large, shallow, well-oiled baking pans (preferably round). Spread with fingers evenly over pan at ¼-inch thickness. Pour on sauce and spread out to ¼-inch from edges. Layer mozzarella on sauce and sprinkle with parmesan. Bake at 400° for 15 to 20 minutes, or until brown and bubbly. Makes 2 pizzas with 8 servings each.

STEP 4: DAY TWENTY-ONE PLAN

For Day Twenty-One, follow your tri-out menu planner from Day Nineteen. At the end of Day Twenty-One, use red ink to circle all planned foods which were not included and to write in any unplanned items you may have eaten. How closely did you approximate your tri-out menu planner for Day Twenty-One? Were any deviations due to unplanned snacking?

The chart on page 162 may help to identify any possible snacking errors. List all snacks eaten on Day Twenty-One and the associated circumstances. Can you pinpoint any areas which require habit modification? If so, you may want to reread Step 2, and refer to the behavior modification suggestions from Day Seventeen. After all, when planned wisely, snacks can provide your diet with essential nutrients, as well as pleasure, variety, and snacking fun!

Day Twenty-One

Snack Food and Amount	Time Snack Began	Ended	Where Eaten*	Body Position†	Hunger Rating‡	Unplanned (✓)	Comments

Notes:
*For example: kitchen table, office, restaurant, car, etc.
†For example: standing at refrigerator, lying on couch, sitting at desk, etc.
‡PH—Physical hunger
 EH—Emotional hunger
 OH—Outside/environmental hunger

DAY TWENTY-TWO

PRACTICAL PLANNING

STEP 1: WEEKLY MENU PLANNING

Daily menu planning is a simple, practical method to ensure the intake of all of your nutrient needs. But daily food shopping would be unnecessarily time-consuming and expensive. Even shopping twice a week can be a hassle. Therefore, advanced planning of a week of meals with accompanying food shopping lists proves more efficient, less costly, and ultimately less wasteful.

On Day Twenty-Two, look at the week of sample menus for Days Twenty-Three through Twenty-Nine on pages 164–169. Explanatory notes are given for each day's menu. Use the menu plan which meets your caloric needs (see Day Sixteen) to devise your own weekly menu planner which suits your personal tastes and individual lifestyle. Be careful in your menu planning so that the alterations you do make in your weekly menu planner, meal pattern, or Nutri-Plan diet plan are beneficial, not detrimental to your personal diet goals. Make your menu goals realistic. Avoid trying to do too much all at once; repeated failure can lead to diet depression and the desire to simply return to old eating patterns. On the other hand, avoid allowing yourself too much leeway: excessive flexibility can lead to undesirable diet deviations, and may ultimately result in overall failure to improve the diet.

Try to create menus which differ from day to day, and include in each day a variety of different foodstuffs. Remember that a well-balanced diet is a varied diet which includes moderate amounts of many different foods. And in planning your menus, be sure to consider the seasons and the types of foods available to you. For example, if blueberries are in season, you may want to include them in several meals or snacks in a variety of forms (eg, on hot cereal, in low-fat yogurt, etc).

Complete another shopping list outliner like the one in Day Nineteen to help you in organizing a shopping list which is coordinated with your weekly menu plan. Foods which you already have on hand need not be included. Remember to add in required seasonings, cleaning products, paper goods, foods for family members, and other items usually purchased in the supermarket but not included in your weekly menu planner.

Proper menu planning utilizing organized shopping lists can be the key to both diet success and supermarket savings.

STEP 2: DAY TWENTY-TWO PLAN

For Day Twenty-Two, follow your tri-out menu planner from Day Nineteen. At the end of Day Twenty-Two, use red ink to circle all planned foods which were not included and to write in any unplanned items you may have eaten. How closely did you approximate your tri-out menu planner for Day Twenty-Two? To what do you attribute any deviations?

It has now been more than three weeks since you began the Nutri-Plan. You are three quarters of the way through! Use the checklist below to indicate (ν) the behavioral changes you have made:

_____ I do not consume an excessive amount of protein.

_____ I do consume a good amount of carbohydrate in the form of starch.

_____ I do not include too much fat in my diet.

_____ I do eat a variety of vitamin-rich foods.

_____ I do eat a variety of mineral-rich foods.

_____ I do include plenty of water in my diet.

_____ My caloric intake approximates that level which I determined to be desirable for me.

_____ I do obtain the recommended number of daily servings from the basic food groups.

_____ I do consume foods which are high in fiber.

_____ I do try to avoid high-fat and high-cholesterol foods.

_____ I do try to avoid foods high in sugar content.

_____ I do try to avoid foods high in salt (sodium) content.

_____ I am moderate in my consumption of alcohol.

_____ My overall diet has improved since Day One.

_____ I consider my diet to be well balanced.

Compare the above list to the one you completed on Day Fifteen. Can you see any improvements since Day Fifteen? And what about behavioral changes since Day Fifteen?

_____ I choose desirable alternatives to food for use as a reward.

_____ I leave one bite on my plate at each meal or snack and resist the temptation to "clean the plate."

_____ I avoid eating due to environmental cues, such as the sight or smell of food.

_____ I avoid fantasizing about food.

_____ I avoid eating according to the clock.

_____ I do make eating a sole activity and avoid eating while engaged in other activities.

_____ I avoid eating in response to emotions, such as tension or boredom.

_____ I avoid eating for the purpose of procrastination.

_____ I seek refuge in places other than the kitchen when people stir up my emotions.

_____ I avoid dissatisfying searches for unknown foods.

_____ I do adhere to my Nutri-Plan diet plan.

_____ I do follow a menu plan.

_____ I do use an organized shopping list.

_____ I do make wise food selections when dining out.

_____ I do make wise snack selections.

In consideration of the amount of dietary change you may have made so far, it is hard to imagine that even more change is possible. The road to good health is not an easy one, but the end results make the journey worthwhile. And improved health through good nutrition is certainly a destination worth traveling toward.

Sample Weekly Menu Planner
(1000 Calorie Nutri-Plan Diet Plan)

Meal	Day Twenty-Three	Day Twenty-Four	Day Twenty-Five	Day Twenty-Six
B R E A K F A S T	½ cup oatmeal with 2 tbsp raisins and ½ cup skim milk	¼ cup granola cereal with ½ cup skim milk 1 sm orange	½ whole wheat English muffin, broiled with ¾ oz part-skim mozzarella ½ cup orange juice	½ cup hot wheat cereal with 2 tbsp raisins and ½ cup skim milk
L U N C H	Tuna openface sandwich: 1 sl cracked wheat bread ¼ cup tuna 2 tsp low-calorie mayo 1 tsp mustard lettuce 1 cup low-fat yogurt with ¼ cup strawberries and ¼ sm banana, sliced	Spinach salad: ¾ cup fresh spinach 1 egg, sliced ¼ cup fresh mushrooms, sliced 1½ oz low-fat cheese, sliced 3 whole rye crackers low-calorie dressing	Chicken salad plate: 1 cup diced chicken 1 tbsp low-calorie mayo herbs and spices lettuce bed ¾ cup strawberries 5 sm gingersnaps	Bagel Broiler—broil: ½ pumpernickel bagel, split with 1 tsp peanut butter and ½ banana, sliced ½ cup skim milk
S U P P E R	3½ oz dry wine 3 oz roast veal ½ cup brown rice with ½ cup sliced mushrooms tossed salad with ½ cup mixed vegetables and low-calorie dressing	3 oz chicken, baked 1 sm potato, baked with ½ tbsp sour cream lettuce hearts with low-calorie Italian dressing ½ cup low-fat yogurt with ½ cup canned pears	3½ oz dry wine Eggplant parmesan—bake: ½ cup steamed eggplant ¼ cup tomato sauce ¼ cup tomatoes, diced herbs and spices —topped with: 2 sliced mushrooms 1½ oz part-skim mozzarella 3 tbsp bread crumbs	4 oz baked fish ½ cup brown rice, cooked with ½ cup sliced zucchini and 20 pistachios, chopped tossed salad with ½ cup mixed vegetables and low-calorie dressing
S N A C K S	1 sm bran muffin ½ cup skim milk	12 oz "light" beer 3 cups popcorn	6 pumpernickel melba toasts ¾ oz part-skim cheese	Homemade nachos—broil: 1 tortilla 1½ oz part-skim mozzarella 12 oz "light" beer

Meal	Day Twenty-Seven	Day Twenty-Eight	Day Twenty-Nine
B R E A K F A S T	¾ cup shredded wheat with ½ sm banana and ½ cup skim milk	½ whole wheat English muffin with 1 egg, poached ½ cup low-fat yogurt with ¾ cup strawberries	½ pumpernickel bagel with 1 tsp peanut butter ½ cup orange juice
L U N C H	Mini pizza—broil: ½ whole wheat English muffin spread with 1 tbsp tomato sauce and 1½ oz part-skim mozzarella ½ cup canned pears	Chef's salad: 1 oz diced turkey 1½ oz low-fat cheese ½ cup mixed vegetables lettuce bed low-calorie dressing 3 arrowroots	Western omelet: 1 egg, beaten with 2 tbsp water ¾ oz part-skim mozzarella ¼ cup diced tomato, onion, pepper, sprouts herbs and spices ½ whole wheat English muffin
S U P P E R	4 oz roast turkey 1 sm sweet potato with 1 tsp margarine ½ cup green beans tossed salad with ½ cup mixed vegetables low-calorie dressing	Hamburger: 2 sl cracked wheat bread 2 oz lean hamburg ½ cup sliced tomato, onion ½ tsp mustard lettuce 12 oz "light" beer	Seafood spaghetti: 1 cup whole wheat spaghetti 3 oz shrimp ½ cup tomato sauce herbs and spices 1 oz grated parmesan cheese tossed salad with ¼ cup sliced mushrooms and low-calorie dressing
S N A C K S	12 oz "light" beer 3 cups popcorn with ½ oz grated parmesan cheese	Banana shake—blend: ½ cup skim milk ½ sm banana 1 tsp vanilla crushed ice	1 sl angelfood cake with ¾ cup strawberries and ½ cup low-fat yogurt

Explanatory Notes

Day	Breakfast	Lunch	Supper	Snacks
Twenty-Three		1 Fat in mayo + ½ Fat in yogurt +	½ Fat in dressing +	1 Fat in muffin
Twenty-Four	1 Fat in granola +	½ Fat in cheese + ½ Fat in dressing + 1 Veg in spinach + 1 Veg in mushrooms No Fruit	¼ Fat in sour cream + ½ Fat in dressing + ¼ Fat in yogurt No Veg 1 Fruit in pears No Luxury	Luxury in beer
Twenty-Five	½ Fat in cheese +	1½ Fat in mayo + 4 Meat in chicken No Grain No Milk Luxury in gingersnaps	½ Fat in cheese + No Meat 1 Grain in breadcrumbs + 1 Milk in cheese + No Luxury	½ Fat in cheese 2 Grain in crackers ½ Milk in cheese
Twenty-Six		No Meat ½ Milk in milk	½ Fat in dressing + 4 Meat in fish No Luxury	½ Fat in cheese 1 Milk in cheese Luxury in beer
Twenty-Seven		No Meat	1 Fat in margarine + ½ Fat in dressing + 4 Meat in turkey No Luxury	½ Fat in cheese Luxury in beer
Twenty-Eight	1 Meat in egg ½ Fat in yogurt +	1 Meat in turkey + ½ Fat in cheese + ½ Fat in dressing + 1 Veg in mixed veg	2 Meat in hamburger 1½ Fat in hamburger 1 Veg in sliced tomato and onion	

Explanatory Notes *(continued)*

Twenty-Nine	1 Fat in peanut butter	¼ Fat in cheese + ½ Veg in vegetables for omelet + No Fruit ½ Milk in cheese	1 Fat in cheese + ½ Fat in dressing + 1 Veg in sauce + ½ Veg in mushrooms 2 Grain in spaghetti + 1 Milk in cheese + No Luxury	¼ Fat in yogurt 1 Fruit in strawberries No Grain ½ Milk in yogurt Luxury in cake

Sample Weekly Menu Planner
(1200 Calorie Nutri-Plan Diet Plan)

Meal	Day Twenty-Three	Day Twenty-Four	Day Twenty-Five	Day Twenty-Six
B R E A K F A S T	½ cup oatmeal with 2 tbsp raisins and ½ cup skim milk	1 cup puffed rice with ¾ cup strawberries and ½ cup skim milk	½ whole wheat English muffin broiled with ¾ oz part-skim mozzarella ½ cup orange juice	½ cup hot wheat cereal with 2 tbsp raisins and ½ cup skim milk
L U N C H	Tuna sandwich: 2 sl cracked wheat bread ¼ cup tuna 2 tsp low-calorie mayo 1 tsp mustard lettuce 1 cup low-fat yogurt with ¼ cup blueberries and ¼ sm banana, sliced	Spinach salad: ¾ cup fresh spinach 1 egg, sliced ¼ cup sliced mushrooms 1½ oz low-fat cheese, sliced low-calorie dressing 4″ sq cornbread	Chicken salad pita sandwich: 1 mini whole wheat pita 1 cup diced chicken 1 tbsp low-calorie mayo herbs and spices lettuce ¾ cup strawberries 5 sm gingersnaps	Bagel Broiler—broil: 1 pumpernickel bagel, split, with 2 tsp peanut butter and ½ sm banana, sliced ½ cup skim milk
S U P P E R	3½ oz dry wine 4 oz roast veal ½ cup brown rice with ½ cup sliced mushrooms tossed salad with ½ cup mixed vegetables and low-calorie dressing ½ fresh apple	4 oz chicken, baked 1 sm potato, baked with ½ tbsp sour cream lettuce hearts with low-calorie Italian dressing ½ cup low-fat yogurt with 1 cup canned pears	3½ oz dry wine Eggplant parmesan—bake: ½ cup steamed eggplant ¼ cup tomato sauce ¼ cup tomatoes, diced herbs and spices—topped with 2 sliced mushrooms 1½ oz part-skim mozzarella 3 tbsp bread crumbs ½ fresh apple	4 oz baked fish ½ cup brown rice ½ cup sliced zucchini tossed salad with ½ cup mixed vegetables and low-calorie dressing ½ sm honeydew melon
S N A C K S	1 sm bran muffin ½ cup skim milk 1 sm orange	12 oz "light" beer 3 cups popcorn with 2 tbsp raisins	Danish bagel—broil: 1 whole wheat bagel, split ¼ cup low-fat cottage cheese ¾ oz part-skim mozzarella nutmeg cinnamon 2 tbsp raisins	Homemade chichen natchos—broil: 1 tortilla 1½ oz part-skim mozzarella 1 oz diced cooked chicken 12 oz "light" beer

Meal	Day Twenty-Seven	Day Twenty-Eight	Day Twenty-Nine
B R E A K F A S T	¾ cup shredded wheat with ½ sm banana and ½ cup skim milk	½ whole wheat English muffin with 1 egg, poached ½ cup low-fat yogurt with ¾ cup strawberries	½ pumpernickel bagel with 1 tsp peanut butter ½ cup orange juice

Meal	Day Twenty-Seven	Day Twenty-Eight	Day Twenty-Nine
L U N C H	Mini pizza—broil: 　1 whole wheat English muffin, 　　split, spread with 　1 tbsp tomato sauce and 　1½ oz part-skim mozzarella ½ fresh pear	Chef's salad: 　2 oz diced turkey 　1½ oz low-fat cheese 　½ cup mixed vegetables 　lettuce bed 　low calorie dressing 1 sm wheat roll	Western omelet: 　1 egg, beaten with 　2 tbsp water 　¾ oz part-skim mozzarella 　¼ cup diced tomato, onion, pepper, 　　sprouts 　herbs and spices 1 whole wheat English muffin
S U P P E R	3½ oz dry wine 3 oz roast turkey 1 sm sweet potato with 　1 tsp margarine ½ cup green beans tossed salad with 　½ cup mixed vegetables and 　low-calorie dressing ½ cup applesauce	Hamburger: 　2 sl cracked wheat bread 　2 oz lean hamburg 　½ cup sliced tomato, onion 　½ tsp mustard 　lettuce 12 oz "light" beer ½ fresh apple	Seafood spaghetti: 　1 cup whole wheat spaghetti 　4 oz shrimp 　½ cup tomato sauce 　herbs and spices 　1 oz grated parmesan cheese tossed salad with 　¼ cup sliced mushrooms and 　low-calorie dressing 2 plums
S N A C K S	Cinnamon-apple broiler—broil: 　½ whole wheat English muffin 　¼ cup low-fat cottage cheese 　½ oz grated cheddar cheese 　½ apple, sliced 　cinnamon	Pear shake—blend: 　½ cup skim milk 　1 cup canned pears 　1 tsp vanilla 　crushed ice	1 sl angelfood cake with 1½ cups strawberries and ½ cup low-fat yogurt

Explanatory Notes

Day	Breakfast	Lunch	Supper	Snacks
Twenty-Three		1 Fat in mayo + ½ Fat in yogurt +	½ Fat in dressing +	1 Fat in muffin
Twenty-Four		½ Fat in cheese + 1 Fat in cornbread + No Fruit 1 Veg in spinach + 1 Veg in mushrooms	¼ Fat in sour cream + ½ Fat in dressing + ¼ Fat in yogurt 2 Fruit in pears No Veg No Luxury	Luxury in beer
Twenty-Five	½ Fat in cheese +	1½ Fat in mayo + 4 Meat in chicken + No Grain Luxury in gingersnaps	½ Fat in cheese + No Meat 1 Grain in bread crumbs + No Luxury	½ Fat in cheese 1 Meat in cottage cheese 2 Grain in bagel
Twenty-Six		2 Fat in peanut butter + No Meat ½ Milk in milk	½ Fat in dressing + 2 Fruit in melon No Luxury	½ Fat in cheese 1 Meat in chicken No Fruit Luxury in beer
Twenty-Seven			1 Fat in margarine + ½ Fat in dressing + 3 Meat in turkey +	½ Fat in cheese 1 Meat in cottage cheese
Twenty-Eight	½ Fat in yogurt + 1 Meat in egg +	1 Fat in cheese + ½ Fat in dressing + 2 Meat in turkey + 1 Grain in roll + 1 Veg in mixed veg + No Fruit	1 Fat in meat 2 Meat in hamburger 2 Grain in bread 1 Veg in tomato, onion	 2 Fruit in pears
Twenty-Nine	1 Fat in peanut butter + No Milk	¼ Fat in cheese + ½ Milk in cheese + ½ Veg in vegs for omelet + No Fruit	1 Fat in cheese + ½ Fat in dressing + 1 Milk in cheese + 1 Veg in sauce + ½ Veg in mushrooms	¼ Fat in yogurt ½ Milk in yogurt + 2 Fruit in strawberries

168

Sample Weekly Menu Planner
(1500 Calorie Nutri-Plan Diet Plan)

Meal	Day Twenty-Three	Day Twenty-Four	Day Twenty-Five	Day Twenty-Six
B R E A K F A S T	½ cup oatmeal with 2 tbsp raisins and ½ sm banana, sliced and ½ cup skim milk	1 cup puffed rice with ¾ cup strawberries and ½ cup skim milk ½ grapefruit	½ whole wheat English muffin broiled with ¾ oz part-skim mozzarella Morning shake—blend: ½ cup orange juice ½ sm banana crushed ice	½ cup hot wheat cereal with 2 tbsp raisins and ½ sm banana, sliced and ½ cup skim milk
L U N C H	Tuna sandwich: 2 sl cracked wheat bread ½ cup tuna 1 tbsp low-calorie mayo 1 tsp mustard lettuce 1 cup low-fat yogurt with ½ cup blueberries and ½ sm banana, sliced	Spinach salad: ¾ cup fresh spinach 1 egg, sliced ¼ cup low-fat cottage cheese ¼ cup sliced mushrooms 1½ oz low-fat cheese, sliced low-calorie dressing 4″ sq cornbread 2 dried apricots	Chicken salad pita sandwich: 1 mini whole wheat pita 1 cup diced chicken 1 tbsp low-calorie mayo herbs and spices lettuce 1½ cups mixed strawberries with 1 tbsp sour cream 5 gingersnaps	Bagel broiler—broil: 1 pumpernickel bagel, split, with 1 tbsp peanut butter ½ sm banana, sliced and 2 dates, chopped ½ cup skim milk
S U P P E R	3½ oz dry wine 4 oz roast veal 1 cup brown rice with ½ cup mushrooms, sautéed in 1 tsp vegetable oil tossed salad with ½ cup mixed vegetables and low-calorie dressing 1 sm apple	4 oz chicken, baked 1 sm potato, baked with 1 tbsp sour cream lettuce hearts with low-calorie Italian dressing ½ cup low-fat yogurt with 1 cup canned pears 3 arrowroots	3½ oz dry wine Eggplant parmesan—bake: ½ cup steamed eggplant ¼ cup tomato sauce ¼ cup tomatoes, diced herbs and spices—topped with: 2 sliced mushrooms 1½ oz part-skim mozzarella 3 tbsp bread crumbs 1 sm wheat roll with 1 tsp margarine 1 sm apple	4 oz baked fish 1 cup brown rice ½ cup sliced zucchini tossed salad with ½ cup mixed vegetables and low-calorie dressing ¼ honeydew melon filled with 10 grapes and 1 tbsp sour cream
S N A C K S	1 sm bran muffin ½ cup skim milk	12 oz "light" beer 3 cups popcorn with 2 tbsp raisins	Danish bagel—broil: 1 whole wheat bagel, split ½ cup low-fat cottage cheese ¾ oz part-skim mozzarella cinnamon nutmeg 2 tbsp raisins	Homemade chicken nachos— broil: 1 tortilla 1½ oz part-skim mozzarella 2 oz diced cooked chicken 12 oz "light" beer

Meal	Day Twenty-Seven	Day Twenty-Eight	Day Twenty-Nine
B R E A K F A S T	¾ cup shredded wheat with ½ sm banana and ½ cup skim milk ½ grapefruit	½ whole wheat English muffin with 1 egg, poached ½ cup low-fat yogurt with ¾ cup strawberries and 2 tbsp raisins	½ pumpernickel bagel with 1 tsp peanut butter and ½ sm banana, sliced ½ cup orange juice
L U N C H	Nutty pizza—broil: 1 whole wheat English muffin split, spread with 1 tbsp tomato sauce 1½ oz part-skim mozzarella 5 walnuts, chopped 1 fresh pear	Chef's salad: 2 oz diced turkey 1½ oz low-fat cheese ½ cup mixed vegetables lettuce bed low-calorie dressing 1 small wheat roll with 1 tsp margarine 4 dried apricots 3 arrowroots	Western omelet: 1 egg, beaten with 2 tbsp water and ¼ cup low-fat cottage cheese ¾ oz part-skim mozzarella ¼ cup sliced tomato, onion, pepper, sprouts herbs and spices 1 whole wheat English muffin with 1 tsp margarine 1 fresh apple

Meal	Day Twenty-Seven	Day Twenty-Eight	Day Twenty-Nine
S U P P E R	3½ oz dry wine 4 oz roast turkey 1 sm sweet potato with 1 tsp margarine ½ cup green beans with 10 almonds, slivered tossed salad with ½ cup mixed vegetables and low-calorie dressing ½ cup applesauce, warmed with 2 tbsp raisins and nutmeg	Hamburger: 2 sl cracked wheat bread 3 oz lean hamburg ½ cup sliced tomato, onion ½ tsp mustard lettuce 12 oz "light" beer ½ sm banana, sliced in 1 tbsp sour cream	Seafood spaghetti: 1 cup whole wheat spaghetti 4 oz shrimp 2–3 sliced mushrooms ½ cup tomato sauce herbs and spices 1 oz grated parmesan cheese tossed salad with low-calorie dressing 3 arrowroots ½ cup applesauce
S N A C K S	Cinnamon-apple broiler—broil: 1 whole wheat English muffin, split ½ cup low-fat cottage cheese ½ oz grated cheddar cheese ½ apple, sliced cinnamon	Pear shake—blend: ½ cup skim milk ½ cup canned pears 1 tsp vanilla crushed ice 3 cups popcorn	1 sl angelfood cake with ¾ cup strawberries and ½ cup low-fat yogurt and 5 almonds, chopped

Explanatory Notes

Day	Breakfast	Lunch	Supper	Snacks
Twenty-Three		1½ Fat in mayo + 1 Fat in yogurt +	1 Fat in oil + 1 Fat in dressing + 2 Fruit in apple	1 Fat in muffin No Fruit
Twenty-Four		1 Fat in cheese + ½ Fat in dressing + 2 Fat in cornbread + 2 Veg in spinach and mushrooms + 1 Fruit in apricots +	½ Fat in sour cream + ½ Fat in dressing + ½ Fat in yogurt ½ Milk in yogurt No Veg 2 Fruit in pears No Luxury	No Milk Luxury in beer
Twenty-Five	½ Fat in cheese	1½ Fat in mayo + ½ Fat in sour cream + 4 Meat in chicken + 1 Grain in pita + No Milk Luxury in gingersnaps	1 Fat in cheese + 1 Fat in margarine + No Meat 1 Grain in bread crumbs + 1 Grain in roll + 1 Milk in cheese + No Luxury	½ Fat in cheese + 2 Meat in cottage cheese 2 Grain in bagel ½ Milk in cheese
Twenty-Six		3 Fat in peanut butter + No Meat ½ Milk in milk +	½ Fat in dressing + ½ Fat in sour cream + 2 Fruit in melon and grapes No Luxury	1 Fat in cheese 2 Meat in chicken 1 Milk in cheese+ No Fruit Luxury in beer
Twenty-Seven		No Meat	1 Fat in margarine + 1 Fat in nuts + 1 Fat in dressing + 4 Meat in turkey + 1 Grain in potato +	½ Fat in cheese 2 Meat in cottage cheese 2 Grain in English muffin
Twenty-Eight	½ Fat in yogurt + 1 Meat in egg +	1 Fat in cheese + ½ Fat in dressing + 1 Fat in margarine + 2 Meat in turkey + 1 Veg in mixed veg +	1½ Fat in beef + ½ Fat in sour cream 3 Meat in beef 1 Veg in sliced tomato, onion	
Twenty-Nine	1 Fat in peanut butter + No Milk	½ Fat in cheese + 1 Fat in margarine + ½ Milk in cheese + ½ Veg in vegs for omelet +	1 Fat in cheese + ½ Fat in dressing + 1 Milk in cheese + 1 Veg in tomato sauce + ½ Veg in mushrooms 2 Grain in spaghetti + 1 Grain in arrowroots	½ Fat in yogurt + ½ Fat in nuts ½ Milk in yogurt No Grain

Weekly Menu Planner
(_____ Calorie Nutri-Plan Diet Plan)

Meal	Day Twenty-Three	Day Twenty-Four	Day Twenty-Five	Day Twenty-Six
B R E A K F A S T				
L U N C H				
S U P P E R				
S N A C K S				

Weekly Menu Planner *(Continued)*
(_____ Calorie Nutri-Plan Diet Plan)

Meal	Day Twenty-Seven	Day Twenty-Eight	Day Twenty-Nine
B R E A K F A S T			
L U N C H			
S U P P E R			
S N A C K S			

DAY TWENTY-THREE

RECOMMENDED RECIPES

STEP 1: REAMS OF RECIPES

You may want to incorporate some of the following nutritious and delicious recipes into your Nutri-Plan diet plan. The calories per serving and approximate number of allowed daily food group servings are given for each recipe. Note that each of these recipes meets some or all of the following criteria:

- Low in fat and cholesterol
- Low in sugar
- Low in sodium
- Low in calories
- High in vitamin and mineral content
- High in fiber content

Moderate amounts of nutrient-rich foodstuffs can serve to further enhance your overall health and well-being. So, enjoy yourself! Eat and be fit!

Breakfast Bargains

Whole Wheat English Muffins—140 calories (2 Grain)

1 pkg dry yeast
½ cup warm water
½ cup skim milk, scalded
½ cup boiling water
1 tbsp honey
2 cups whole wheat flour
1 cup all-purpose flour
½ cup unprocessed bran
1 tsp salt
½ tsp soda
12 tuna cans, 6½ oz
cornmeal

Dissolve yeast in warm water. Mix milk and boiling water together in large bowl. Add honey to milk mixture and let stand until lukewarm. Stir in yeast and whole wheat flour. Cover with damp cloth and let sit in warm area until doubled in bulk. Punch down.

Combine next four ingredients and blend into dough. Turn out onto floured board and knead well. Return to bowl, cover, and let rise again for 25 to 30 minutes.

Remove both ends of tuna cans, wash well, remove labels, and oil insides. Punch down dough and roll out to ½ inch thickness. Cut into circles with tuna cans and transfer to a flat surface. Let rise in cans for an hour or until doubled. Dust both sides of circles with cornmeal. Toast on an ungreased griddle, until browned on both sides (about 6 to 8 minutes). Remove cans after first side browns—rings are hot, so be careful. Cool muffins on a rack, then split into halves with a fork. Toast just prior to serving. Makes 1 dozen muffins.

◆

Fruit Crunch Muffin—145 calories (½ Fruit + 1 Grain + ½ Meat)

½ whole wheat English muffin
2 tbsp cottage cheese, uncreamed
1 tbsp applesauce, unsweetened
1 tbsp raisins
1 tbsp wheat germ
¼ tsp cinnamon
¼ tsp nutmeg

Blend together cheese, applesauce, raisins and wheat germ and spread on muffin half. Sprinkle with cinnamon and nutmeg and broil until bubbly. Serve hot. Serves one.

◆

Cream Cheese Crunch Spread—25 calories (½ Fruit)

1 tbsp cream cheese
2 tbsp low-fat yogurt
1 tbsp wheat germ
1 tbsp raisins
1 tbsp dried unsweetened coconut

Blend together and chill. Makes 6 (1 tbsp) servings. Spread on whole grain bagels, toast, or English muffins.

Crunchy Granola Cereal—110 calories (1 Grain + 1 Fat)

4 cups rolled oats
1 cup wheat germ
¼ cup chopped walnuts
¼ cup slivered almonds
2 tbsp sesame seeds
2 tbsp raisins
2 tbsp dates, chopped
2 tbsp dried coconut
2 tbsp unprocessed bran
¼ cup honey
¼ cup vegetable oil
½ cup water

Combine all but last three ingredients thoroughly and spread evenly in bottom of large baking pan. Blend together last three ingredients and heat slightly. Pour over dry mixture and combine thoroughly. Heat slowly at 225° for 2 hours. Turn with a spatula every 15 minutes. Store in refrigerator. Makes 28 (¼ cup) servings.

◆

Apple-Cinnamon French Toast—125 calories (½ Fruit + 1 Grain + ¼ Meat)

1 egg, beaten with 1 egg white
¼ cup skim milk
¼ tsp vanilla extract
4 sl whole wheat bread, halved
1 cup applesauce, unsweetened
dash cinnamon
dash nutmeg

Mix egg, milk and vanilla together. Soak bread in mixture for 3 minutes, turning once. Brown egg-bread in non-stick pan over medium heat. Warm applesauce in saucepan with spices. Top each bread half with ¼ cup warm sauce and serve immediately. Serves 4.

◆

Whole Wheat Waffles—135 calories (1 Grain + 1 Fat)

1¼ cups whole wheat flour
¼ cup wheat germ
1 tsp salt
2 tsp baking powder
2 eggs, separated
1½ cups skim milk
3 tbsp vegetable oil
2 tbsp honey

Preheat waffle iron. Stir together dry ingredients. Beat yolks well. In separate bowl, beat whites until stiff peaks form. Add milk, oil and honey to yolks and blend well. Stir into dry mixture. Fold in egg whites and pour into waffle iron. Makes 10 waffles.

◆

Baked Pancake—130 calories (1 Grain + 1 Fat)

2 tbsp margarine
1½ cups skim milk
1 cup whole wheat flour
1 tbsp honey
¾ tsp cardamom
⅛ tsp salt
3 eggs

Melt margarine in a 2×8×14-inch baking dish in 400° preheated oven. Mix remaining ingredients together and pour into baking dish. Bake about 30 minutes, or until golden brown and puffy. Serve at once. Makes 8 servings. Delicious with unsweetened applesauce, berries, peach slices, or sliced bananas.

◆

Bubbly Fruit Broil—100 calories (½ Fruit + 1 Meat + ½ Fat)

½ cup cottage cheese, uncreamed
¼ cup pineapple chunks, unsweetened
1 tbsp raisins
1 tbsp chopped walnuts
¼ cantaloupe, 5″ dia
dash cinnamon

Mix cheese, pineapple and raisins together. Add walnuts. Scoop mixture into melon and top with cinnamon. Broil 2 to 3 minutes or until bubbly. Serves two.

Light 'N Luscious Luncheons

All luncheon recipes make one serving unless otherwise noted. Caloric values for salad recipes include dressings.

Chef's Salad—220 calories (2 Veg + 1 Milk + 1 Meat + 1 Fat)

1 cup lettuce, in bite-size pieces
1 tomato, in wedges
¼ green pepper, thinly sliced
¼ cup red cabbage, shredded
2 radishes, sliced
1 oz cooked chicken or turkey, in strips
1 oz part-skim cheese, in strips
sprouts

Combine vegetables in salad bowl. Arrange strips of meat and cheese on top of vegetables. Sprinkle with sprouts and serve with 1 tbsp Chef's dressing.

◆

Seafood Salad—160 calories (2 Veg + 2 Meat)

1 cup lettuce, in bite-size pieces
½ cucumber, thinly sliced
3 cherry tomatoes, halved

¼ green pepper, thinly sliced
1 tbsp onion, minced
1 tbsp parsley, chopped
5 lg cooked shrimp
¼ cup crabmeat
1 tbsp grated parmesan cheese
dash paprika

Combine vegetables in salad bowl. Arrange shellfish on vegetables. Sprinkle with cheese and paprika and serve with 2 tbsp Seafood Dressing.

◆

Spinach Salad—210 calories (2 Veg + 1 Meat + 1½ Fat)

⅓ lb fresh spinach, in bite-size pieces
4 mushrooms, halved
1 scallion, chopped fine
¼ cup waterchestnuts
1 egg, hard boiled
1 tbsp slivered almonds

Combine vegetables in salad bowl. Separate cooked egg, discard yolk, and chop white. Sprinkle salad with egg, nuts and Wheaty Croutons. Serve with 1 tbsp Spinach Salad Dressing.

◆

Wheaty Croutons—25 calories (¼ Grain)

1 tbsp vegetable oil
4 sl whole wheat bread, cut in ¼" squares
1 tbsp wheat germ
¼ tsp garlic powder
¼ tsp onion powder
dash oregano
dash soy sauce

Combine all ingredients and stir until each cube is well coated. Spread on foil-lined baking sheet and broil for 10 minutes, or until golden brown. Makes 16 (1 tbsp) servings.

◆

Health Salad—215 calories (2 Veg + ½ Fruit + 1 Meat + 2 Fat)

1 cup lettuce, in bite-size pieces
¼ sm carrot, grated
½ sm tomato, in wedges
¼ green pepper, thinly sliced
1 stalk celery, chopped
¼ sm cucumber, thinly sliced
1 tbsp sesame seeds
1 tbsp chopped walnuts
1 tbsp raisins
¼ cup cottage cheese, uncreamed
sprouts

Combine vegetables in salad bowl and sprinkle with seeds, walnuts and raisins. Mound cottage cheese on top and garnish with sprouts. Serve with 1 tbsp Health Dressing.

◆

Vegetable Plate I—85 calories (2 Meat)

½ cup cottage cheese, uncreamed
2 tbsp skim milk
1 tbsp parsley, chopped
1 tsp chopped chives
1 tbsp low-calorie bleu cheese dressing

Blend thoroughly in blender. Sprinkle with paprika and chill. Serve with assorted raw vegetables.

◆

Vegetable Plate II—85 calories (½ Milk + ½ Fat)

½ cup low-fat yogurt
2 tbsp skim milk
1 tbsp parsley, chopped
1 tsp chopped chives
1 tbsp low-calorie bleu cheese dressing

Blend thoroughly in blender. Sprinkle with paprika and chill. Serve with assorted raw vegetables.

◆

Whole Wheat Mini Pitas—70 calories (1 Grain)

1½ tsp dry yeast
1 cup water, warm
1 tbsp honey
1½ cups whole wheat flour
1½ cups all-purpose flour
1½ tsp salt

Dissolve yeast in water with 1 tsp honey and let stand 5 minutes. Add remaining honey, flour and salt. Mix well with wooden spoon. Knead 10 minutes and place in lightly oiled bowl. Cover with a cloth and let rise for 1½ hours in a warm place. Punch down, knead for 2 minutes, divide into 20 equal portions. Form each into a smooth, round ball. Cover with a cloth and let stand for 15 minutes. Preheat oven to 475°. Roll out each ball with a rolling pin to ½" thickness. Place on foil-lined baking sheets and bake on lower rack in oven for 10 minutes, or until puffed and brown. Wrap each in a towel and place in a paper bag for 15 minutes, or until deflated without cracking. Makes 20 Mini Pitas.

◆

Tuna Pita Bake—275 calories (1 Grain + 1 Milk + 1 Meat + 1½ Fat)

¼ cup tuna fish, drained and flaked
1 tbsp celery, chopped
1 tbsp onion, minced
1 tbsp green pepper, chopped
1 tbsp carrot, grated
dash garlic powder
dash pepper
2 tsp low-calorie mayonnaise
1½ oz part-skim mozzarella cheese

Mix together all ingredients except cheese and stuff into whole wheat mini pita. Top tuna with cheese and close pita sandwich. Wrap in foil and bake at 350° for 15 minutes. Check to see that cheese is melted and serve immediately.

◆

Tuna Broiler—270 calories (1 Grain + 1 Milk + 1 Meat + 1½ Fat)

1 sl rye bread
¼ cup tuna
1 tbsp celery, chopped
1 tbsp onion, chopped
1 tbsp green pepper, chopped
1 tbsp carrot, chopped
dash garlic powder
dash pepper
2 tsp low-calorie mayonnaise
1½ oz part-skim mozzarella cheese
lettuce, shredded
sprouts

Mix tuna, vegetables, seasonings and mayonnaise together and spread evenly on bread. Top sandwich with cheese and broil until bubbly. Serve topped with lettuce and sprouts.

◆

Yogurt-Cheese Melt—215 calories (1 Grain + 1 Milk + ½ Fat)

2 tbsp low-fat yogurt
1 tbsp green pepper, finely chopped
1 tsp wheat germ
dash garlic powder
dash pepper
½ whole wheat English muffin
1½ oz part-skim mozzarella cheese, in strips
dash grated parmesan cheese
lettuce, shredded

Mix yogurt, green pepper, wheat germ and seasonings thoroughly and chill. Arrange cheese strips on muffin. Spread on yogurt mixture and sprinkle with parmesan cheese. Broil until bubbly. Top with lettuce and serve immediately.

◆

Bagel-Pizza—140 calories (1 Grain, + ½ Milk + ¼ Fat)

1 pumpernickel bagel
¼ tsp mustard
¾ oz part-skim mozzarella cheese, in strips
2 sl tomato
2 mushrooms, sliced
dash oregano
dash pepper
dash parmesan cheese

Dot bagel half with mustard and layer with cheese, tomato, and mushrooms. Sprinkle seasonings and parmesan cheese onto bagels and broil until cheese is bubbly. Serve hot.

◆

Good Ol' Peanut Butter—135 calories (½ Fruit + 1 Grain + 1 Fat)

1 sl cracked wheat bread
1 tsp peanut butter
½ sm banana, sliced
1 tsp dried unsweetened coconut

Spread bread with peanut butter. Top with banana and sprinkle with coconut. Broil until browned and bubbly. Serve at once.

Deluxe Dinners

Herbed Halibut—175 calories (3 Meat)

1 lb halibut (or other firm-fleshed fish)
½ tsp herbed salt
⅛ tsp basil
⅛ tsp marjoram
⅛ tsp parsley flakes
½ cup dry white wine
1½ tbsp lemon juice
1 tbsp whole wheat flour
¾ cup mushrooms, chopped fine
½ cup grated low-fat cheese

Place filets in a casserole dish. Mix seasonings into wine and lemon juice. Pour over fish and marinate in refrigerator for at least 30 minutes. Drain off liquid and thicken slightly with flour over low heat. Stir in mushrooms and cheese, and spread over fish. Bake at 400° for 25 minutes or until sauce bubbles. Serves 4.

◆

Popover Sole Roll—160 calories (2 Meat +1 Fat)

3 large fillets of sole
1 lemon, sliced
dash pepper
2 tsp margarine
¼ cup dry white wine

Sauce
2 tbsp margarine
2 tbsp whole wheat flour
¾ cup skim milk
⅓ cup dry sherry
1 tsp dill weed
1 tsp parsley flakes
dash pepper

Wash fish and pat dry. Split each in half lengthwise and rub with lemon. Place with skin side down, dot with pepper, and roll up. Stand rolls in glass pie plate or casserole dish, dot with margarine, and pour wine over all. Bake uncovered at 350° for 20 minutes, basting several times.
Sauce: Heat margarine in small sauce pan, add flour and cook over medium heat until bubbly, stirring constantly. Reduce heat and gradually add milk, stirring with wire whisk until thickened and

smooth. Remove from heat. Add sherry, 3 tbsp liquid from fish, and seasonings. Remove tops from popovers (see below) and fit sole rolls into bottom halves of popovers. Pour ½ cup sauce into each, sprinkle with paprika, and replace top. Serve warm. Makes 6 servings.

◆

Whole Wheat Popovers—135 calories (1 Grain + 1 Fat)

2 eggs
1 cup skim milk
1 tbsp vegetable oil
½ cup all-purpose flour
½ cup whole wheat flour
½ tsp salt

Beat eggs, add milk and oil. Mix dry ingredients together, add to egg mixture, and beat with wooden spoon until smooth. Fill paper-lined muffin tins half full and bake at 400° for 35 minutes, or until puffy and brown. Makes 6 popovers.

◆

Fish Florentine—225 calories (1 Veg + 3 Meat + 1 Fat)

10 oz pkg frozen chopped spinach
1 tbsp margarine
½ cup onion, chopped fine
2 tbsp whole wheat flour
½ cup skim milk
½ cup dry white wine
1 lb fresh white fish, 4 fillets
(flounder, halibut, haddock, or sole)
½ lb fresh mushrooms, sliced
1 tbsp margarine
dash parsley flakes
dash paprika

Cook spinach according to package directions and drain well. Melt margarine in large skillet and sauté onions until tender. Add flour and cook 2 minutes, stirring constantly. Gradually add milk and bring to a boil; add wine and heat until thickened, stirring constantly. Add ¼ cup sauce to spinach. Place 2 tbsp spinach on each fillet and roll up. Place in foil-lined baking pan, seam-side down. Sauté mushrooms in margarine and add to remaining sauce. Pour over fish rolls and bake at 350° for 15 minutes, or until tender. Sprinkle parsley and paprika on fish and serve. Serves 4.

◆

Scallop K-Bob—195 calories (1 Veg + ½ Fruit + 3 Meat)

1 lb sea scallops
8 oz can pineapple chunks, unsweetened
¼ cup lemon juice
⅛ cup soy sauce
⅛ cup dry white wine
12 mushroom caps
12 cherry tomatoes
sm green pepper, in 1" squares
2 tsp vegetable oil

Drain juice from pineapple and reserve chunks. Combine liquids and marinate scallops, cover and refrigerate for an hour. Baste occasionally. Drain liquid and reserve. Thread scallops on long skewers alternately with vegetables and pineapple chunks. Brush with reserved marinade, then oil. Broil 10 minutes, turning once, or until scallops are cooked and tender; continue to brush with marinade while cooking. Serves 4.

◆

Chicken Bake—205 calories (3 Meat)

2 lb chicken, roaster
1 lg onion, thinly sliced
2 med carrots, thinly sliced
1 lg clove garlic, minced
1 cup dry white wine
½ tsp rosemary
½ tsp thyme
¼ tsp salt
⅛ tsp pepper

Place chicken in large casserole and add remaining ingredients. Cover and bake at 400° for 1¼ hours, or until chicken is tender. Drain liquid and serve hot. Serves 6.

◆

Roast Chicken—210 calories (3 Meat)

2 lb chicken, roaster
1 med onion, chopped
3 carrots, halved
2 cloves garlic, minced
¼ tsp cumin
⅛ tsp salt
juice of lemon

Place chicken in a roasting pan and spread onion and carrots around it. Sprinkle with seasonings and lemon juice. Cover and roast at 450° for 1 hour, or until chicken is tender. Serves 6.

◆

Herbed Chicken—190 calories (3 Meat)

2 lb chicken, roaster
¾ tsp sage
½ tsp thyme
½ tsp marjoram
½ tsp dry mustard
4 bay leaves
dash pepper

Place chicken in large casserole and sprinkle with seasonings. Bake at 450° for 45 minutes. Reduce to 375° and continue baking for 10 to 15 minutes, or until chicken is tender. Serves 6.

◆

Chicken Continental—280 calories (3 Meat + 1 Fat)

¼ cup lemon juice
⅓ cup dry white wine
1 clove garlic, minced
¼ tsp thyme
2½ lb chicken, broiler or fryer
2 tbsp margarine
dash pepper

Mix lemon juice, wine, garlic, and thyme together. Place chicken in large pie plate and cover with marinade. Refrigerate 1 to 2 hours, basting occasionally. Cut chicken into serving pieces and arrange in a single layer in foil-lined baking dish. Dot with margarine, sprinkle with pepper, and bake at 425° for one hour, or until fork tender, turning once. Serves 6.

◆

Chicken Divine—250 calories (1 Veg + 2 Meat + 1 Fat)

1½ lb chicken, fryer or broiler
1 tsp margarine
dash oregano
dash pepper
1 cup fresh mushrooms, sliced
1 tsp margarine
10 oz pkg broccoli, frozen

Sauce
3 tbsp margarine
3 tbsp whole wheat flour
1 cup chicken broth
1 tsp dill weed
1 tsp tarragon
dash garlic powder

1 tbsp parsley flakes
2 tbsp wheat germ
2 tbsp grated parmesan cheese

Place chicken in foil-lined baking dish, dot with margarine, season, and bake at 350° for 20 to 25 minutes, or until done. Cool; remove skin and bone. Sauté mushrooms in margarine in heavy skillet and reserve. Cook broccoli according to package directions, drain well, and place evenly in bottom of shallow baking dish.

Sauce: Heat margarine in saucepan, add flour, and cook briefly over medium heat. Blend in broth slowly, stirring constantly, until thickened and smooth. Stir in mushrooms (including any liquid) and seasonings.

Top broccoli with chicken slices and pour mushroom sauce over all. Sprinkle with parsley, wheat germ, and cheese. Bake uncovered at 375° for 20 minutes, or until brown and bubbly on top. Serves 6.

◆

Lean Lamb Italiano—200 calories (2 Veg + 2 Meat + 1 Fat)

6 lean lamb chops, loin cut
1 tbsp vegetable oil
1 tsp garlic, chopped fine
½ tsp oregano
¼ tsp thyme
½ bay leaf
½ cup dry red wine
1 cup tomatoes, pureed in blender, mixed with
1 tbsp tomato paste
1 tsp vegetable oil
1 cup green pepper, thinly sliced
½ lb fresh mushrooms, sliced

Trim fat and broil chops 2 to 3 minutes, turning once to brown on both sides. Drain on paper towel and pat off excess fat. Cook garlic and herbs in oil in large skillet for 30 seconds, stirring constantly. Add wine and boil briskly, stirring to scrape bottom of pan. Stir in tomatoes and tomato paste and add chops. Baste, cover, and simmer over low heat for 1 hour, or until meat is tender. Heat 1 tsp vegetable oil in small skillet and cook pepper until tender. Add mushrooms and cook 2 minutes longer. Drain and add to chop mixture. Cover, simmer 5 minutes, then simmer uncovered for 10 minutes or until sauce is thickened. Serve at once. Serves 6.

◆

Lamb K-Bobs—210 calories (2 Veg + 2 Meat + 1½ Fat)

3 tbsp vegetable oil
3 tbsp lemon juice
¼ cup dry sherry
2 tsp soy sauce
1 tsp garlic powder
½ tsp rosemary
¼ tsp pepper
2 sm onions, chopped fine
1½ lb lean lamb, cut in cubes
18 cherry tomatoes
18 mushroom caps
18 onion wedges, 1″ square
18 green pepper wedges, 1″ square

Mix first eight ingredients together to make marinade. Place lamb cubes in shallow glass pan, cover with marinade, and refrigerate overnight. Drain and reserve marinade. Thread meat and vegetables evenly onto 8 skewers. Broil or grill for 15 minutes, turning once; baste occasionally with marinade. Serves 6.

◆

Seasoned Beef Roast—275 calories (3 Meat + 3 Fat)

2½ lbs beef roast
1 cup dry red wine
½ tsp thyme

1 tsp lemon juice
1 tbsp vegetable oil

Preheat oven to 350°. Place roast in large foil-lined baking pan. Mix remaining ingredients and use to baste roast. Bake 1½ to 2½ hours, until cooked as desired. Serves 10.

Herbed Veal Roast—200 calories (3 Meat + ½ Fat)

3 lb rolled rump veal roast
2 tbsp margarine
¼ tsp salt
½ tsp pepper
½ tsp rosemary
1 cup dry red wine

Brown veal briefly in margarine. Season veal, place in roasting pan, and pour wine over all. Roast at 400° for 2 hours, or until veal is tender. Serves 12.

Veal 'n Eggplant Parmigiana—300 calories (2 Veg + ¼ Milk + 2 Meat + 2 Fat)

1 tbsp vegetable oil
1 sm onion, chopped
½ green pepper, chopped
3 cups tomato puree
1 sm can tomato paste
1 tbsp oregano
1 tsp basil
1 tsp garlic powder
1 clove garlic, minced
1 tbsp vegetable oil
1 egg, beaten with 1 egg white
2 tbsp skim milk
1 lb very lean, thin veal cutlets
1 med eggplant, peeled, cut in ½" thick slices
wheat germ
¼ cup dry wine
6 oz part-skim mozzarella cheese, thinly sliced
3 tbsp grated parmesan cheese

Heat 1 tbsp oil in large skillet. Add onion and pepper; saute until slightly brown. Pour off excess oil, add tomatoes and season with oregano, basil and garlic powder. Cover pan, lower heat, and simmer for 1 hour or more.

In large skillet, brown garlic clove in 1 tbsp oil. Remove visible garlic pieces. Beat egg and milk together in shallow dish. Dip veal in egg, then wheat germ, and brown in garlic-oil 5 minutes on each side. Drain on paper towel, patting to absorb oil. Repeat with eggplant, browning for 3 minutes on each side, and drain well on paper towel. Stir wine into tomato sauce and simmer 5 more minutes. Cover bottom of casserole dish with ¼ cup sauce. Alternate veal and eggplant in layers, topping each layer with mozzarella slices and covering with sauce. Pour remaining sauce over top, sprinkle with parmesan, and bake at 350° until cheese is bubbly. Serves 8.

Peppery Stuff—200 calories (2 Veg + ½ Grain + 2 Meat + 3 Fat)

1¼ cups tomato puree, mixed with
1 sm can tomato paste
1 tbsp oregano
1 tsp basil
1 tsp garlic powder
6 lg green peppers
1 tbsp vegetable oil
½ med onion, chopped
¼ cup mushrooms, sliced
2 tbsp celery, chopped
½ lb lean ground beef
¾ cup cooked brown rice
3 tbsp chopped walnuts
1 tbsp parsley flakes
¼ tsp thyme
¼ cup skim milk
½ tsp basil
¼ cup chicken broth
½ cup low-fat yogurt
3 tbsp grated parmesan cheese

Simmer tomato mixture with oregano, basil, and garlic powder in saucepan for at least 1 hour. Cut ¼" slice from top of each pepper and remove seeds. Cover with boiling water and cook 5 minutes; drain.

Heat oil in large skillet and sauté vegetables until slightly browned. Add meat and cook 5 minutes, until meat is browned. Remove from heat and drain off excess fat. Add rice, walnuts, parsley, thyme and milk to meat mixture and blend thoroughly with fork. Fill peppers and arrange in deep baking dish.

Combine basil and chicken broth with tomato sauce, bring to a boil, and remove from heat. Pour over and around peppers, cover dish tightly, and bake at 400° for 45 minutes or until peppers are tender but crisp. Baste several times while baking. Remove peppers from oven and top each with yogurt. Sprinkle with cheese and return to oven for 2 to 3 minutes, until yogurt begins to melt. Serve hot. Serves 3 (2 each).

Refried Tortillas—380 calories (1 Veg + 2 Grain + ½ Milk + 1 Meat + 2½ Fat)

1½ cups kidney beans
5 cups water

Soak beans in water overnight. Drain well.

½ cup onion, chopped
¼ cup tomato, chopped

¼ tsp garlic powder
1 tsp chili powder
dash cayenne pepper

Cook with beans until beans are soft.

2 tbsp vegetable oil
½ cup onion, chopped
½ tsp garlic, minced

Sauté until onions are transparent.

¾ cup tomato, chopped

Add to onions and cook 3 minutes. Mash spoonful of bean mixture into vegetable mixture with a fork until well bended. Continue to add bean mixture by spoonfuls, mashing after each addition. When all is mixed, cook for 10 minutes more, turn off heat, and cover.

1 cup onions, chopped fine
1 tsp oregano
½ tsp garlic, minced
⅛ cup vinegar
dash tabasco

Combine in small bowl, mix thoroughly and reserve.

2 tbsp vegetable oil
2 tbsp vinegar
1 tsp soy sauce
3 cups lettuce, shredded

Combine oil with vinegar. Add soy sauce and drop in lettuce. Toss until well coated.

12 sm corn tortillas, frozen
12 tbsp grated parmesan cheese

Bake tortillas according to package directions until crisp. Sprinkle each with ¼ cup bean mixture. Top each with ¼ cup lettuce mixture, 2 tbsp tabasco mixture, and 1 tbsp cheese. Serve at once. Serves 6 (2 each).

◆

Cheese Tortillas—370 calories (2 Veg + 1 Grain + 1½ Milk + 2 Fat)

6 med tomatoes, chopped
1 cup onions, chopped fine
1 tsp oregano
½ tsp garlic, minced
½ cup vinegar
dash tabasco

Combine in small bowl, mix thoroughly, and chill.

2 tbsp vegetable oil

2 tbsp vinegar
1 tsp soy sauce
3 cups lettuce, shredded

Combine oil with vinegar. Add soy sauce and drop in lettuce. Toss until well coated.

12 sm corn tortillas, frozen
9 oz part-skim mozzarella cheese

Bake tortillas according to package directions until crisp. Top each with ¾ oz cheese and return to oven until cheese melts.

2 med tomatoes, chopped
1 sm green pepper, chopped
1 sm onion, chopped
1 cup low-fat yogurt
½ cup cottage cheese, uncreamed
1 tbsp low-calorie mayonnaise
1 tbsp mustard
dash soy sauce

Mix together. Spread 2 tbsp on each cheese-topped tortilla and return to oven until bubbling hot.

12 tbsp grated parmesan cheese

Top each tortilla with ¼ cup lettuce mixture, 2 tbsp tabasco mixture, and 1 tbsp cheese. Serve at once. Serves 6 (2 each).

◆

Cheesey Spinach Squares—285 calories (1 Veg + ½ Milk + 2 Meat + 2 Fat)

3 (10 oz) pkg frozen chopped spinach
3 tbsp margarine
¾ lb fresh mushrooms, sliced
6 eggs
1½ cups soft whole wheat bread cubes
1 tbsp Worcestershire sauce
2 eggs
2 cups cottage cheese, uncreamed
dash soy sauce
6 tbsp grated parmesan cheese

Cook spinach according to package directions and drain well. Melt margarine in large skillet and sauté mushrooms until tender. In large bowl, beat 6 eggs. Add bread cubes, Worcestershire, spinach, and mushrooms. Mix well.

Beat two eggs in medium bowl; add cottage cheese and soy sauce and mix well. Spread half of spinach mixture in pan, cover with cottage cheese mixture, and top with remaining spinach mixture. Bake uncovered at 350° for 30 minutes, or until knife comes out clean when inserted in center. Refrigerate until cool, then cut into squares. Top each with 1 tbsp parmesan cheese and serve cold or rewarmed. Serves 6.

◆

Spinach Pasta Bake—305 calories (½ Veg + 1 Grain + ½ Milk + 1 Meat + 3 Fat)

10 oz pkg frozen chopped spinach
2 tbsp margarine
2 tbsp whole wheat flour
½ tsp oregano
¼ tsp onion powder
dash pepper
dash soy sauce
½ cup part-skim cheese, shredded
1 cup low-fat yogurt
2 tbsp sour cream
1½ cups spinach noodles, cooked
1 cup cottage cheese, uncreamed
3 tbsp wheat germ
3 tbsp grated parmesan cheese

Cook spinach in saucepan until slightly limp. Puree in blender and reserve. Melt margarine, stir in flour with wire whisk, and cook 2 minutes, stirring constantly. Add spinach puree and cook 3 minutes, stirring frequently. Add seasonings and part-skim cheese. Stir in yogurt and sour cream; continue to whisk for 1 minute. Remove from heat.

Place half of noodles in casserole. Top with half of spinach mixture. Spread with cottage cheese, remaining noodles, then remaining spinach. Sprinkle wheat germ and parmesan cheese over top and bake uncovered at 350° for 30 minutes, or until bubbling hot. Serve warm. Serves 4.

◆

Whole Wheat Macaroni 'n Cheese—230 calories (1 Grain + 1 Milk + 1½ Fat)

2 quarts water
2 cups whole wheat macaroni
2 tbsp margarine
2 tbsp whole wheat flour
2 cups skim milk
1 tsp garlic powder
dash pepper
dash paprika
2 eggs, slightly beaten
1 cup low-fat cheese, shredded
2 tbsp wheat germ

Bring water to boil, drop in macaroni, and cook 7 minutes or until tender. Drain well. Heat margarine in saucepan and stir in flour; cook 2 minutes and gradually add milk, stirring constantly. Add seasonings and continue to stir over medium heat until thickened and smooth. Remove from heat and cool slightly. Add eggs to sauce and mix well.

In casserole dish, arrange layers of macaroni, sauce, and cheese. Top with sprinkling of wheat germ. Bake 15 to 20 minutes at 375° until brown and bubbly. Makes 6 (⅔ cup) servings.

◆

Chinese Vegetables—275 calories (1 Veg + 1 Grain + 1 Milk + 2 Fat)

1 cup broccoli cuts
½ cup green beans
½ onion, thinly sliced
½ cup mushrooms, sliced
¼ cup red cabbage, thinly sliced
¼ cup waterchestnuts
¼ cup bamboo shoots
¼ cup pea pods
2 tbsp soy sauce
2 tbsp dry white wine
2 tbsp vegetable oil
1 tbsp slivered almonds
2 cups brown rice, cooked
9 oz part-skim mozzarella cheese, shredded

Combine vegetables, soy sauce, and wine in large skillet and stir-fry in oil until tender-crisp. Toss almonds with vegetables. Toss hot, cooked rice with cheese. Top with stir-fried vegetables and serve immediately. Makes 6 (⅔ cup) servings.

◆

Fluffed Carrots—95 calories (2 Veg + 1 Fat)

12 carrots, halved
2 tbsp margarine
1 tsp lemon juice
¼ tsp cinnamon
¼ tsp nutmeg
1 tbsp parsley flakes

Wash and peel carrots. Place in saucepan, cover with water, and bring to boil. Cover and simmer until tender. Drain well and mash. Add margarine, lemon juice, cinnamon and nutmeg to mashed carrots and mix well. Sprinkle parsley on carrots and serve. Serves 6.

◆

Crunchy Carrot Salad—70 calories (½ Fruit + ½ Veg + 1 Fat)

2 cups carrots, shredded
½ cup seedless raisins
¼ cup low-calorie mayonnaise
¼ cup low-fat yogurt
2 tbsp lemon juice
dash salt

Combine carrots and raisins in salad bowl. Blend remaining ingredients together and pour over carrot mixture. Mix well and chill. Makes 8 (¼ cup) servings.

◆

Coleslaw De-light—55 calories (1 Veg + ½ Fat)

2 tbsp honey
⅔ cup vinegar
2 tbsp vegetable oil
½ tsp salt

½ tsp pepper
dash soy sauce
2 lb cabbage, shredded
1 med onion, chopped
1 lg carrot, shredded

Combine honey, vinegar and oil well. Mix seasonings and soy sauce into honey mixture. Mix vegetables in large bowl. Pour dressing over all and toss to mix. Cover and refrigerate several hours before serving. Makes 16 (½ cup) servings.

◆

Stir-fry Broccoli—80 calories (1 Veg + 1 Fat)

2 tbsp vegetable oil
¾ lb broccoli, chopped
1¼ cups mushrooms, sliced
1 large carrot, cut in strips
1 clove garlic
½ tsp salt
¼ tsp thyme
¼ tsp sesame seeds

Heat oil in skillet over medium heat. Add rest and cook, stirring constantly, for 5 to 8 minutes or until vegetables are tender-crisp. Makes 6 (½ cup) servings.

◆

Sesame Zucchini—55 calories (1 Veg + 1 Fat)

1 tbsp vegetable oil
1 tbsp onion, chopped
1 clove garlic, minced
½ tsp rosemary
2 cups zucchini, thinly sliced
1 tbsp sesame seeds
dash soy sauce

Heat oil in large skillet, add onion, garlic and rosemary and cook until onion is transparent. Add remaining ingredients to onion and continue cooking, stirring occasionally, until tender-crisp. Makes 4 (½ cup) servings.

◆

Cheese-Baked Cauliflower—125 calories (1 Veg + ½ Milk + 1½ Fat)

3 cups cauliflower pieces
3 tbsp margarine
3 tbsp whole wheat flour
2 cups skim milk
1 cup part-skim cheese, shredded
1 tbsp dry white wine
½ tsp dry mustard
dash soy sauce
dash tabasco sauce
2 tbsp parmesan cheese
dash paprika

Cook cauliflower in small amount of water until tender-crisp. Place in casserole dish.

Melt margarine in saucepan and stir in flour with wire whisk. Cook for 2 minutes, stirring constantly. Add milk gradually, lower heat, and continue stirring until smooth and thickened. Add cheese, wine, mustard, soy and tabasco sauces and mix well. Pour over cauliflower. Sprinkle parmesan cheese and paprika over top and bake at 350° for 20 minutes until bubbly. Makes 8 (½ cup) servings.

◆

Cheese Baked Potatoes—90 calories (1 Grain)

6 sm baking potatoes
½ cup cottage cheese, uncreamed
1 tbsp onion, minced
¼ tsp garlic powder
1 tbsp grated parmesan cheese
1 additional tbsp grated parmesan cheese
dash paprika

Preheat oven to 425°. Wash, dry, and fork-prick potatoes. Bake for 1 hour, or until done. Cut a slice from the top of each, scoop out cooked potato pulp, and mash.

Whip next four ingredients in blender until creamy. Blend enough into mashed potato pulp to make a light, fluffy mixture. Spoon back into potato skins in smooth mounds. Place potatoes on foil-lined baking sheets, sprinkle tops lightly with parmesan cheese and paprika, and return to oven until lightly browned. Serves 6.

◆

Spiced Rice—140 calories (1 Grain + 1 Fat)

2½ cups water
1 cup brown rice
3 sm onions, chopped fine
½ cup mushrooms, sliced
1 tbsp margarine
¼ tsp basil
¼ tsp garlic powder
¼ tsp savory
2 tbsp grated parmesan cheese
1 tbsp parsley flakes

Bring water to boil. Add rice, cover, and simmer 40 minutes, or until all water is absorbed. Sauté vegetables in margarine and add basil, garlic, and savory. Cook 2 minutes, then pour over warm rice. Sprinkle parmesan cheese and parsley onto rice and mix lightly with a fork. Makes 6 (½ cup) servings.

◆

Rice Almondine—125 calories (½ Grain + 1 Fat)

1½ cups brown rice
2 tbsp margarine
½ cup slivered almonds
1 tsp salt

3 cups water

Combine all in heavy saucepan. Bring to boil, cover tightly, and simmer without stirring for 35 minutes or until liquid has evaporated. Makes 12 (¼ cup) servings.

◆

Rice with Vegetables—130 calories (1 Veg + 1 Grain + ½ Fat)

2 tbsp margarine
1 med onion, chopped
2 cups zucchini, thinly sliced
1 cup corn niblets
1 cup tomatoes, chopped
3 cups brown rice, cooked
¼ tsp oregano
¼ tsp salt
⅛ tsp pepper

Sauté zucchini and onion in margarine in large skillet until barely tender. Add remaining ingredients, cover and simmer 10 to 15 minutes until warmed. Makes 9 (¾ cup) servings.

◆

Bulgur Wheat Pilaf—115 calories (1 Grain + ½ Fat)

1½ tbsp vegetable oil
1 carrot, diced
1 stalk celery, diced
⅓ cup mushrooms, sliced
1 bay leaf
1¾ cup water
1 cup raw bulgur wheat
½ tsp salt

Heat oil in heavy pot, add vegetables and bay leaf, and cook over medium heat for 3 minutes. Add water to vegetables, bring to a boil, cover and simmer 5 minutes. Add bulgur wheat and salt and bring to a rapid boil. Cook over low heat, covered, for 15 minutes. Uncover, and simmer until liquid is evaporated. Makes 8 (½ cup) servings.

◆

Kasha—155 calories (2 Grain + ½ Fat)

1 cup dry buckwheat groats
1 egg, lightly beaten
2 cups boiling water
2 tbsp margarine
¼ tsp salt
⅛ tsp pepper

Stir first three ingredients together and place in hot skillet. Cook over high heat, stirring constantly, until the grains are separate and dry. Stir in margarine and seasonings, cover tightly, and steam over low heat for 30 minutes. Makes 8 (½ cup) servings.

◆

Polenta—190 calories (1 Grain + 2 Fat)

6 cups water
2 cups cornmeal
¼ tsp salt
¼ cup margarine
½ cup grated parmesan cheese

In a large pot, bring water to a boil and pour corn meal in slowly, stirring constantly. Add salt and margarine to cornmeal and cook slowly over low heat for 2 to 3 minutes, stirring frequently with a wooden spoon. When mixture is thick and smooth, stir in cheese and cook for a few more minutes. Makes 8 (½ cup) servings.

Dazzling Dressings

Chef's Dressing—16 calories/tbsp (½ Fat)

¾ cup dry red wine
1 tsp vegetable oil
1 tsp vinegar
1 clove garlic, minced
1 tsp oregano

Combine all in jar and shake well. Chill. Store in refrigerator. Makes ¾ cup.

◆

Seafood Dressing—25 calories/tbsp (½ Fat)

1 cup low-fat yogurt
1 cup low-calorie mayonnaise
½ cup chili sauce
2 tbsp lemon juice
1 tbsp onion, minced
¼ tsp tarragon
dash tabasco sauce
dash pepper

Combine all in large bowl and mix well. Store in jar under refrigeration. Makes 2¾ cups.

◆

Spinach Salad Dressing—20 calories/tbsp (½ Fat)

⅓ cup low-calorie mayonnaise
¼ cup lemon juice
¼ cup cold water
2 tbsp grated parmesan cheese
1 clove garlic, minced
dash pepper
dash soy sauce

Combine all in jar and shake well. Chill. Store in refrigerator. Makes 1 cup.

◆

Health Dressing—23 calories/tbsp (½ Fat)

½ cup low-calorie mayonnaise
½ cup low-fat yogurt
1 tbsp sesame seed

1 tbsp honey
dash cinnamon

Combine all in large bowl and mix well. Chill. Store in jar in refrigerator. Makes 1 cup.

◆

Low-Calorie Bleu Cheese Dressing—10 calories/tbsp (unlimited)

1 cup cottage cheese, uncreamed
⅓ cup buttermilk
1 tbsp bleu cheese
dash pepper

Combine all in blender and mix until creamy and smooth. Chill. Store in refrigerator. Makes 1⅓ cups.

◆

Low-Calorie French Dressing—10 calories/tbsp (unlimited)

1 cup cottage cheese, uncreamed
⅓ cup buttermilk
1 tsp paprika
¼ tsp dry mustard
dash onion powder
dash garlic powder
dash Worcestershire sauce
1 to 2 tbsp tomato juice

Combine all but tomato juice in blender and mix until creamy and smooth. Thin to desired consistency with tomato juice. Chill. Store in refrigerator. Makes 1⅓ cups.

◆

Low-Calorie Creamy Italian Dressing—17 calories/tbsp (½ Fat)

¼ cup low-calorie mayonnaise
¼ cup vinegar
¼ cup cold water
½ tsp oregano
dash garlic powder
dash onion powder
dash paprika

Combine all in jar and shake well. Chill. Store in refrigerator. Makes ¾ cup.

◆

Avocado-Lite Dressing—23 calories/tbsp (½ Fat)

1 ripe avocado, peeled and pitted
¼ cup skim milk
6 tbsp low-fat yogurt
1 tbsp vinegar
1 clove garlic, minced
dash soy sauce

Combine in blender and mix until smooth. Chill. Store in refrigerator. Makes 1¼ cups.

◆

Vinaigrette—12 calories/tbsp (unlimited)

¾ cup dry white wine
1 tsp vegetable oil
1 tsp vinegar
1 clove garlic, minced
1 tbsp onion, minced
1 tsp oregano

Combine all in jar and shake well. Chill. Store in refrigerator. Makes ¾ cup.

◆

Next to Nothing Dressing—8 calories/tbsp (unlimited)

1 cup cottage cheese, uncreamed
⅓ cup buttermilk
¼ tsp dry mustard
1 tbsp onion, minced
1 tbsp parsley flakes
1 tbsp chopped chives
1 tsp dill weed

Combine all in blender and mix until creamy and smooth. Chill. Store in refrigerator. Makes 1⅓ cups.

Super Sauces

Special Sour Cream—8 calories/tbsp (unlimited)

1 cup cottage cheese, uncreamed
½ cup low-fat yogurt
2 tbsp lemon juice
dash pepper
dash salt

Combine in blender and mix until smooth. Chill. Store in refrigerator. Makes 1½ cups.

◆

Special Seafood Sauce—22 calories/tbsp (½ Fat)

½ cup low-fat yogurt
½ cup low-calorie mayonnaise
¼ cup chili sauce
1 tbsp lemon juice
1 tbsp onion, minced
1 tsp horseradish
dash pepper
dash tarragon
dash garlic powder

Combine all in jar, cover, and shake well. Chill. Store in refrigerator. Makes 1¼ cups.

◆

Hot Sauce—25 calories/tbsp (½ Fat)

1 clove garlic, minced
1 med onion, chopped
2 tbsp vegetable oil
¼ cup lemon juice

½ tsp oregano
½ tsp cumin
¼ tsp curry
¼ tsp thyme
dash tabasco sauce
dash Worcestershire sauce
1 cup tomato sauce

Sauté garlic and onion in vegetable oil for 2 to 3 minutes. Add remaining ingredients to onion mixture and simmer 15 to 20 minutes. Chill. Makes 1 cup.

◆

Simple Tomato Sauce—10 calories/tbsp (unlimited)

1 sm onion, chopped
2 cloves garlic, minced
1 tbsp vegetable oil
8 medium tomatoes, chopped
1 tsp tarragon
1 tsp oregano
1 tsp parsley flakes
½ tsp salt
dash pepper
1 cup dry white wine

Sauté onion and garlic in vegetable oil until onions are golden. Add tomatoes and seasonings to onions and cook over medium heat, stirring constantly. Stir wine into sauce and simmer for ½ hour. Add more wine if liquid is needed. Serve immediately or store in refrigerator. Makes 3 to 4 cups.

◆

Vanilla Sauce—35 calories/tbsp (½ Luxury)

⅓ cup honey
1½ tbsp whole wheat flour
2 tbsp margarine, melted
1 cup water
2 tbsp vanilla

Stir honey, flour and margarine together. Add water and cook over low heat, stirring constantly until thickened. Remove from heat and stir in vanilla. Serve over fruit. Makes 1 cup.

◆

Nut Creme—50 calories/tbsp (1 Fat)

1 cup almonds, chopped
2 to 3 tbsp pineapple juice
dash cinnamon
dash nutmeg

Blend in blender until smooth and creamy. Serve on baked apples or other fruit. Makes ½ cup.

◆

Lively Libations

Pineapple Slim Shake—135 calories (1 Fruit + 1 Milk)

1 cup skim milk
½ cup pineapple chunks
1 tsp vanilla
crushed ice

Blend in blender until frothy. Serve immediately. Serves one.

◆

Berry Slim Shake—145 calories (1 Fruit + 1 Milk)

1 cup skim milk
¾ cup strawberries or
½ cup raspberries or
½ cup blueberries or
½ cup combination
1 tsp honey
crushed ice

Blend in blender until frothy. Serve immediately. Serves one.

◆

Banana 'n Date Slim Shake—175 calories (2 Fruit + 1 Milk)

1 cup skim milk
½ sm banana, sliced
2 dates
1 tsp vanilla
crushed ice

Blend in blender until frothy. Serve immediately. Serves one.

◆

Buttermilk Orange Drink—95 calories (1 Fruit + ½ Milk)

2 cups buttermilk
2 cups orange juice
1 tbsp honey

Stir together and chill. Makes 4 (1 cup) servings.

◆

Yogurt Cocktail—55 calories (1 Veg + ¼ Milk)

1 cup low-fat yogurt, plain
2 cups tomato juice
¼ tsp salt
¼ tsp caraway seed
1 tsp onion, chopped fine

Blend in blender. Add 2 ice cubes and blend again. Serve at once. Makes 4 (1 cup) servings.

◆

*Spiced Tea—0 calories (unlimited)

Flavored tea
dash cinnamon
dash cloves, ground

Prepare tea and let set with spices for at least 10. minutes.

◆

*Herbed Tea—0 calories (unlimited)

4 tsp herbs
1 quart boiling water

Add a combination of your favorite herbs to boiling water. Let stand until it reaches strength you desire. Strain. Keep refrigerated, and serve cold or hot.

◆

Hot Molasses Drink—135 calories (1 Milk)

1 cup hot skim milk
1 tbsp molasses
cinnamon stick

Stir molasses into milk. Serve in a mug with cinnamon stick stirrer. Serves one.

◆

Club Soda Cooler—25 calories (½ Fruit)

¾ cup club soda
¼ cup orange juice or

---

*Beware of dangerous herbs (see Day Twenty-Seven).

¼ cup grapefruit juice or
3 tbsp pineapple juice
orange or pineapple slice

Pour liquids into a tall frosted glass. Garnish with fruit slice. Serves one.

◆

Tropical Cooler—115 calories (2 Fruit)

1 lemon, peeled
1 grapefruit, peeled
1 orange, peeled
4 tbsp honey
½ cup mashed papaya
¾ cup water
crushed ice

Blend in blender until frothy. Freeze or serve at once. Watch out for seeds! Makes 4 (1 cup) servings.

STEP 2: DAY TWENTY-THREE PLAN

On Day Twenty-Three, revise your weekly menu planner to include some of the recommended recipes which appeal to you. (Do not forget to revise your shopping list outliner from Day Twenty-Two as well.) Which recipes did you include on Day Twenty-Three? Were they as delicious as they are nutritious?

Your Revised
Weekly Menu Planner
(_____ Calorie Nutri-Plan Diet Plan)

Meal	Day Twenty-Three	Day Twenty-Four	Day Twenty-Five	Day Twenty-Six
B R E A K F A S T				
L U N C H				
S U P P E R				
S N A C K S				

188

Meal	Day Twenty-Seven	Day Twenty-Eight	Day Twenty-Nine
B R E A K F A S T			
L U N C H			
S U P P E R			
S N A C K S			

Shopping List Outliner
For Weekly Menu Planner

Food	Amount
Fruit	
Vegetables	
Grains	
Milk and Cheese	

Food (continued)	Amount
Meat	
Alternates	
Fats	
Beverages	
Luxury	
Miscellaneous	

DAY TWENTY-FOUR

GOING TOO FAR

STEP 1: NEVER TOO THIN?

With the current emphasis on and interest in weight loss, the opposite problem—being too thin—seems to have been forgotten. Yet, there are many Americans, especially women, who are far too thin; and the creed of the beautiful people: "You can never be too thin or too rich" has never been more apparent than in America today.

Due to the desire for a slender body, many people, especially adolescent females, undertake extreme means of weight reduction. Although the best body weight is one which affords "comfort" (as measured by efficiency, health, and general appearance), social acceptance often takes precedence. Some people actually sacrifice everything, including good health, for a thin figure.

It is part of the American temperament to believe in miracles, and fad diets are popular miracles to have faith in. Ever since we have been made acutely aware of the dangers of being overweight, a journalistic frenzy of books on fad diets has appeared in the marketplace. The constant bombardment of information on fast "crash" diets, which promise dramatic results almost overnight, has confused many people about the nutritional implications of such dietary regimes. Young women especially are aware of body weight, yet are unaware of the female physiology which steadily increases female body fat during puberty.

All too often, the uninformed public tries popular fad diets in an effort to achieve the greatest effect in the shortest possible time. Essential foods and a balanced diet are ignored in the quest for lowered body weight.

Reflect on your diet history and try to answer (✓) the questions listed below as honestly as possible. Have you ever:

Yes No
☐ ☐ Undertaken a "crash" diet?
☐ ☐ Fasted in order to lose weight?
☐ ☐ Continued to diet upon reaching your desired weight?
☐ ☐ Become ill due to excessive dieting?

☐ ☐ Felt fat, while others warned that you were too thin?
☐ ☐ Become underweight due to excessive dieting?
☐ ☐ Been at a weight 20% or more below your desired weight?
☐ ☐ Been diagnosed as having "anorexia nervosa"?

What is "anorexia nervosa"? If you answered Yes to more than half of the above questions, you may want to find out more about anorexia nervosa, and identify your own anorexic tendencies. You may also want to consider the dietary habits of your friends, your own children, and any female adolescents with whom you are acquainted, as you learn more about anorexia nervosa.

STEP 2: ANOREXIC TENDENCIES

Which of the following factors do you think might cause an individual to voluntarily starve him or herself for an extended period of time:

☐ biological predisposition to develop such a disorder
☐ genetic predisposition to develop such a disorder
☐ hormonal influences
☐ environmental influences (eg, family relationships, early feeding patterns, and familial attitudes about food)
☐ societal pressures to be thin, with an overemphasis on weight loss dieting

Anorexia nervosa, or self-imposed starvation, is believed to have multiple causes, including one or more of these factors. A pernicious disorder, anorexia nervosa is a syndrome which primarily occurs in adolescent females shortly after the onset of puberty. Teased by friends or family, or overly self-conscious about body contours, susceptible individuals become painfully weight conscious and resolutely begin on regimens of semi-starvation. During this time, the body emits some warning signals:

- the empty stomach churns and growls.
- the blood sugar level drops, causing weakness, fatigue, and trembling.
- reduced fluid intake forces kidneys to concentrate the urine.
- lack of bulk leads to constipation.

As semi-starvation continues, some individuals lose their appetites, while for others control over the urge to eat becomes an all-absorbing concern. Fear of overweight results in food phobias and total avoidance of most foods, lest temptation be too great and lead to overeating.

Many of these chronic dieters are never really overweight to begin with. In fact, the adolescent female may have just begun to adjust "baby fat" and round out her newly developing figure. Yet, the importance of being thin and the dread of obesity become a total preoccupation, as often occurs with those who have successfully lost weight. Dieting may continue toward the goal of size three, when a size nine may be more appropriate in terms of natural build.

The anorexic continues to starve, going beyond simple weight loss and remaining on a semi-starvation regimen until protein-calorie malnutrition and clinical vitamin or mineral deficiencies develop. Anorexics become dangerously obsessed with dieting and weight loss. Some die.

Thus, figure-conscious individuals, most often adolescent females, actually undertake life-threatening diets in search of thinness. Is being one of the "beautiful people" worth the accompanying health damages, and the possibility of death from starvation?

STEP 3: ANOREXIA NERVOSA DIAGNOSED

For the list below, indicate (✔) which health problems you think could be associated with anorexia nervosa:

_____ nutritional deficiencies
_____ lowered resistance to infection
_____ delayed recovery from illness
_____ slowed wound healing
_____ heartbeat pattern alterations
_____ circulatory disorders
_____ hormonal disturbances

Although there is no specific laboratory test for anorexia nervosa, clinical findings and laboratory results can indicate any of the above health concerns in the anorexic. Early diagnosis is essential to prevent physical, psychological and overall health breakdown. Once weight loss is well advanced, however, diagnosis is relatively simple and treatment is a matter of life and death.

In addition to marked weight loss, physical symptoms of anorexia include:

- dry skin and hair
- cold hands and feet
- slowed heartbeat
- low blood pressure
- growth of lanugo hair (fine body hairs)
- diminished sweating
- cold intolerance
- cessation of menstruation

Oftentimes, the anorexic will have episodes of overeating, followed by self-induced vomiting. Anorexics may also resort to diuretics and laxatives to further weight loss. These practices can result in:

- erosion of tooth enamel
- dehydration
- vitamin and mineral deficiencies

Anorexics have a neurotic aversion to food, rather than a physical loss of appetite. Poor physical health is only one result of excessive, unbalanced dieting. Anorexics may display extreme personality changes, often becoming nervous, self-conscious, and hypersensitive to criticism. Other psychological signs associated with anorexia nervosa include:

- irritability
- compulsiveness
- striving for perfection
- withdrawal from social interests
- excessive daydreaming
- physical overactivity, hyperactiveness

The following traits are also typical of the anorexic:

- Despite extreme emaciation, does not consider self as too thin.
- Despite prolonged starvation, denies hunger.
- Despite vigorous and often ritualized exercise (to further weight loss), denies fatigue.

Thus, the desire for a physically thin appearance can result in health deterioration and psychological impairment. Yet, as long as our excessive social preoccupation with the thin look continues to exist, potential anorexics will regard good health as only a secondary concern.

STEP 4: BODY IMAGES

Although most dieters do not have the emaciated appearance of the true anorexic, some do exhibit compulsive tendencies regarding food and diet. Dieters often become compulsive about their eating habits and obsessed with weight loss. It is also common for a dieter to develop an altered self-image and a distorted view of his or her own body; after losing weight, an individual may still see him/herself as fat. Some people prior to weight loss—and even normal-weight individuals—consider themselves to look far fatter than they really are. And, of course, the opposite alteration is also common, in which the self-image is far thinner than the physical self.

What is your body image? Do you think that you see yourself as others see you? You may want to try the following activity in order to determine how closely your body image approximates physical reality. Choose an honest* partner to assist you. You'll need two pencils, three large sheets of unlined paper, and a full-length mirror.

1) Sketch your body shape as you think you look; outline your figure as simply, yet realistically, as you possibly can. At the same time, have your partner sketch you as he or she sees you. Do not look at your partner's drawing.
2) Look at yourself in a full-length mirror for several minutes.
3) While still in front of the mirror, outline your body shape as you now see it.
4) Compare all three sketches. Did you draw yourself differently after you looked in the mirror? Do either of your own sketches resemble your partner's? Do you think that you may be perceiving yourself as fatter or thinner than you actually appear?

You may need to work at altering your own body image, especially if your weight is currently in transition.

STEP 5: ANOREXIA IN ACTION

The following letter, received in 1974 by the Nutrition Department at Harvard's School of Public Health, illustrates the thought processes of the typical victim of anorexia nervosa:

Dept. of Nutrition
Harvard University
Cambridge, Mass. 02138

Dear Mr. F.J. Stare, MD, PhD:

Hi! I know I really should not be bothering a busy man, such as yourself, but I want some

---

*Make sure that your partner can really be honest with you, and will not simply try to bolster your confidence or feed your ego.

answers—and I am hoping you will give them to me. My name is Joanne and right now I am a sophomore in college, majoring in Physical Therapy. To get straight to the point, I feel I have a weight problem—I am not terribly overweight, but I cannot keep my weight constant. I have been watching my diet for over two-and-one-half years now. Before that I was not actually fat—just stocky—my highest weight was between 120 and 125. I am 5'4¼"—I played sports in high school (hockey, basketball, softball, and swimming) and I have been very active throughout my whole life, both in recreational and work activities. Anyway, in my senior year of high school I became concerned about what I ate instead of eating anything when I was hungry—ie, pizza, fried foods, starches, desserts, etc. I was never a compulsive eater or anything, but I ate my share of snacks and soft drinks at parties and all. Well, I evaluated my eating habits and changed them—I have not had a soft drink, fried food, and the like in the last two years. (I must admit though that when I drink an alcoholic beverage I do use diet cola.) Everything was fine, I lost 20 pounds in two months and maintained it well—until I left for college in September of 1972. I went to the University of Florida where I had myself on a strict budget—I spent less than ten dollars per month on all expenses—foods, cards, toiletries, etc. Therefore, I was not eating very nutritiously. I lived on dry cereal, dry milk, cottage cheese, jello, and fresh fruit. I went home at Christmas time weighing 90 pounds.

Then my body went blah—my menstrual periods stopped, and I retained water, which in turn made me feel fat. I became concerned and ate less to compensate. Nobody, including me, understood how I functioned as well as I did on such a diet—my roommate said I was like a plant. Oh, sometimes I felt like my legs would not lift anymore, but I would just convince myself I could do it, and I usually did.

Well, I had told my doctor at home and he performed tests, but it took him until November of 1973 to find out what was wrong, mainly because he did not believe me—in fact he was convinced I was pregnant, but what's really ironic is that I am incapable of pregnancy at this time. Obviously, the biggest problem was psychological acceptance—and I have accepted it for now because I am not really ready for a family anyway. But they did put me on estrogen pills, to retain my female characteristics, and the pills caused me to gain more weight. I was used to weighing between 100 and 105; now I weigh about 115 pounds (with a teeshirt and gym trunks, early in the morning). I do not like that—I am not comfortable. I talked to my family doctor and he said it is from the pills and that I am not fat—and he dropped it: Boom! But I can't. I am uncomfortable and feel blah! My eating habits were bad nutritiously for awhile, so when I thought about it—maybe it is possible I messed up my metabolism without the proper nutrition. I have read all kinds of things on the proper things to eat and I decided to eat two or three balanced meals a day with lowered calories and carbohydrates. Right now I am eating about 300 to 800 calories per day—I enclose my food consumption for the past month (I keep track). This has been the most I ate in the past year or so. I am still active, I jog about two to three miles per day, bike, exercise, swim, sit in the sauna, compete in judo, and participate in judo and jujitsu, while going to college and working. I realize this is a long, detailed letter, but I am hoping you will bear with me and help me, I must be doing something wrong or else something serious is wrong with me physically. Thank you very much—I will be waiting for your reply.

Sincerely,
Joanne

- weight may be temporarily lost, only to be rapidly reacquired.
- undesirable eating habits remain unchanged or become even less supportive of good health.
- anorexia nervosa or bulimia develop, with its health-damaging and life-threatening side effects.

Try to maintain an accurate body image. Whenever you glance in a mirror, take a few minutes to really look at yourself. This is especially important if you are in the process of losing weight; be careful not to become a fat person inside a thin body.

Unwise dieting practices can prove equally, or perhaps even more, dangerous than excess weight. Remember, a wise diet is an essential foundation block in building yourself a long and healthy life. Why shake your own foundation?

STEP 6: DAY TWENTY-FOUR PLAN

For Day Twenty-Four, continue to follow your weekly menu planner from Day Twenty-Two. Try to include some of the smart snacks and recommended recipes from Days Twenty-One and Twenty-Three. At the end of Day Twenty-Four use red ink to circle all planned foods which were not included and to write in any unplanned items you may have eaten. How closely did you approximate your weekly menu planner for Day Twenty-Four? To what do you attribute any deviations? Do you find yourself excluding too many foods? Are you cutting out essentials in order to cut down on calories? Are you trying to speed up your weight loss rate?

Be careful to avoid the temptation to alter your Nutri-Plan diet plan. Do not change it into a fad diet or "crash" diet plan. Nutritional deficiencies, health damages, and the hazards of anorexia nervosa could result.

Wise selection of a variety of foods in moderate amounts will help to support nutritional and physical health. Immoderacy in either direction— that is, too little or too much—can have serious implications and lifelong effects on your physical and psychological health. Just as it is detrimental to yield to the temptation to overeat, it is equally unwise and unhealthy to succumb to the urge to "crash" diet for quick results. Drastic restriction of food intake inevitably results in failure because:

Joanne's Food Consumption for One Month

Sunday/March 24*	Monday/March 25	Tuesday/March 26	Wednesday/March 27

8 AM Tea
  1 tbsp peanut butter
  4 pcs melba toast
1:30 PM ½ breast chicken
  1 tbsp cottage cheese
  2 gl water
	8 AM 1 sl bread with cheese
	  Tea
	2 PM bowl tomato soup
	  6 Ritz crackers
	  2 sl chicken
	  1 gl skim milk
		8 AM 2 eggs, 1 sl bacon
		  Tea
		12 PM 4 sl cheese
		6 PM 1 meatloaf sandwich
		  1 tbsp Rice-A-Roni
		  1 tbsp cottage cheese
		  1 gl skim milk
			8 AM 4 pcs melba toast
			  1 tbsp peanut butter
			2:30 PM apple
			5 PM ½ meatloaf sandwich
			  1 tbsp cottage cheese

Thursday/March 28	**Friday/March 29**	**Saturday/March 30**	**Sunday/March 31**

7:30 AM 2 eggs with cheese
  2 slices bacon
  2 cups tea
12:30 PM 6 choc chip cookies
6 PM 2 hot dogs
  1 tbsp cottage cheese
  1 gl skim milk
	10 AM Apple
	1 PM 1 pc cheese
	8 PM 1 slice steak
	  1 tbsp corn
	  2 pcs bread
	  2 gl brandy
		10 AM 2 eggs with cheese
		  1 cup tea
		8:30 PM 1 sl steak
		  1 tbsp corn
		  2 pcs bread
		  4 gl wine
		  ½ cup strawberries
			Red wine
			4 PM 1 hot choc
			6 PM 2 pcs cheese
			  1 pc bologna

Monday/April 1	**Tuesday/April 2**	**Wednesday/April 3**	**Thursday/April 4**

8:30 AM Bowl Rice Krispies,
  skim milk, ½ cup strawberries
5:30 PM 1 can Slender Chocolate
  Milk Drink (S.C.)
	7:30 AM 1 can S.C.
	11 AM Apple, 1 pc cheese
	6 PM can S.C., 1 pc cheese
	10 PM 1 cup tea
		9 AM can S.C.
		11:15 AM 1 pc cheese
		6:30 PM can S.C.
		10:30 PM 1 cup tea
			7:30 AM gl S.C., apple
			3 PM can S.C., orange
			6:30 PM Bowl of corn flakes,
			  skim milk

Friday/April 5	**Saturday/April 6**	**Sunday/April 7**	**Monday/April 8**

7:30 AM gl S.C.
11:30 AM 2 hard-boiled eggs
5 PM can S.C.
	8 AM can S.C.
	  6 Ritz crackers
	8 PM 2 pcs of cheese
	  10 Ritz crackers
	  2 cups tea
	8:30 PM 1 Cheese Whopper (with
	  only ketchup), carton of milk
		8:30 AM 6 strawberries
		3 PM 1 orange
		  2 cups coffee
		  6 pretzels
		9:30 PM 1 sl steak
		  1 tbsp cottage cheese
		  1 tbsp corn
		  4 strawberries
		  1 gl skim milk
			8:30 AM 1 can S.C.
			  1 pc cheese
			3 PM 1 cup strawberries
			  2 pcs cheese
			6:30 PM 1 can S.C.
			  2 pcs cheese
			  1 cup tea

Tuesday/April 9	**Wednesday/April 10**	**Thursday/April 11**	**Friday/April 12**

7:30 AM 1 cup tea
  2 pcs cheese
1 PM 2 pcs cheese, 10 crackers
  1 orange, 1 cup tea
6:30 PM 1 can S.C.
  6 crackers, 1 pc cheese
7:30 PM 1 cup tea
  2 crackers
	9:30 AM 1 can S.C.
	  1 pc cheese
	11:30 AM 1 orange
	  1 cup corn flakes
	6 PM 1 can S.C.
		7:30 AM 1 orange
		  1 pc cheese
		4:30 PM 1 can S.C.
		  1 pc cheese
			3 PM Cheese and crackers
			  1 gl skim milk

Saturday/April 13	**Sunday/April 14**	**Monday/April 15**	**Tuesday/April 16**

2:30 PM 3 gl wine
  1 sl steak
  1 pc bread
  1 dish applesauce
  2 pcs celery
	11 AM 2 pickles
	3 PM 2 gl wine
	  2 pcs turkey
	  1 pat jelly
	  gravy
	  1 tbsp cottage cheese
	  1 pc ice cream cake
	  (2) 7&7 drinks
		8 AM 1 cup tea
		  4 strawberries
		10:30 AM 1 pc celery
		5:30 PM 1 hamburger
		  1 pc cheese
		  1 tbsp cottage cheese
		  1 cup sl diet peaches
		  1 gl skim milk
			7:30 AM Bowl of puffed rice,
			  skim milk
			  1 orange
			2 PM 1 celery stick
			  2 pcs cheese
			6:30 PM 2 broiled hot dogs,
			  mustard
			  1 bowl diet fruit cocktail
			  1 gl skim milk

Wednesday/April 17	**Thursday/April 18**	**Friday/April 19**	

9 AM Bowl puffed rice, skim milk
  1 orange
  2 hard-boiled eggs
  1 cup Alba 66
5:30 PM 1 can S.C.
  ½ cup cottage cheese
	7:30 AM Bowl of puffed rice, milk
	  1 orange
	1 PM ½ cup cottage cheese,
	  bowl diet peaches
	6:30 PM 1 can S.C.
		9:30 AM 1 pickled egg
		  1 pc bread with cheese
		  1 cup tea
		6:30 PM 6 strawberries
		  1 pc cheese
		  2 pretzels	

*I use "Sweet 'N Low" instead of sugar; I don't salt anything; I broil everything; and I use all "diet" food (ie, margarine, fruit, milk, cheese).

DAY TWENTY-FIVE

ADDING IN ACTIVITY

STEP 1: WHY EXERT YOURSELF?

The importance of regular physical exercise in control of body weight and maintenance of overall health is too often ignored. It is far easier to avoid exercise than it is to recognize the importance of altering a sedentary lifestyle. Do you view exercise as:

- hard work?
- boring?
- time consuming?
- sweat producing?
- dull and repetitious?
- simply no fun?

Or, do you consider exercise as:

- a psychological lift?
- good for your heart and lungs?
- muscle toning?
- a good way to use up calories?
- good, clean fun?

Much research now indicates that it is not just our current patterns of overeating but, more importantly, under-exercising which has led to the ever-increasing percentage of overweight Americans. More and more evidence is accumulating to support the many possible health benefits believed to be associated with regular physical exercise.

Indicate (✓) whether you think the following statements are True or False:

True	False	
☐	☐	Exercise increases the appetite of the sedentary individual.
☐	☐	The amount of energy (calories) used during exercise is so small that unreasonable amounts of exercise time are required for weight loss to result.
☐	☐	Regular physical exercise would be too difficult to incorporate into your lifestyle.

The above statements are three popular myths about exercise. By explaining and exploring these common fallacies, you can choose to adopt an individualized exercise program which suits your particular lifestyle.

STEP 2: BENEFITS OF REGULAR EXERCISE

There is no question that anyone who is involved in daily strenuous physical activity requires more calories than does a sedentary individual. Yet, if a typically sedentary individual adopts a regular program of physical exercise, appetite will actually decrease. This is due to certain complex physiological mechanisms which result in signals to the brain to shut off the appetite. Exercise can also affect psychological outlook, so that feeling physically fit replaces the urge to overeat with the desire to eat low-calorie, high-nutrient foods. Thus, a program of regular physical activity can help to diminish appetite, and can be used to fill a segment of time when undesirable eating behaviors typically occur. After all, if you are running, swimming, or playing tennis, you probably will be too busy to feel hungry—and it is also most likely that you will not be eating at the same time.

Regular physical exercise will provide you with the following health benefits:

- strengthened cardiovascular system—heartbeat becomes stronger, pulse is steadier, blood pressure lowers, and overall circulation improves.
- improved muscle endurance—built up gradually with increased muscle load, recovery from exercise becomes faster and duration of exercise periods can be lengthened.
- increased muscle strength—exercised muscles become stronger with better endurance levels; digestion improves.
- increased flexibility—muscles become stretchable and supple.
- improved coordination—endurance, strength,

and flexibility combine with a sense of balance to make body movement more efficient.

Some additional health benefits that can result from regular physical exercise include:

- improved functioning of lungs
- improved muscle tone
- weight loss
- reduction in chronic fatigue
- improved sleeping patterns
- decrease in tension
- decrease in depression
- improved self-confidence
- improved sex life

Which of the above self-improvements would you like to make? Are the above health benefits worth a bit of sweat and strain? Once you see how easy it is to incorporate an exercise program into your lifestyle—and knowing the health benefits which inevitably result—you probably will not hesitate to make physical activity a regular part of your daily life.

STEP 3: EAT 'N RUN

Many people, especially the overweight, are under the false assumption that exercise does not assist in weight loss. Many believe that the amount of exercise required to utilize 3500 calories—and thereby lose one pound—makes exercise a nearly useless ordeal. The chart below further illustrates this misconception. After all, who would walk six miles for a Big Mac?

Food and Amount	Calories	No. Minutes of Exercise to Utilize the Calories*
apple, 1 sm	50	20 min stroll or 7 min brisk walk
apple pie, lg slice	350	140 min stroll or 50 min brisk walk
skim milk, 12 oz	100	10 min jog or 5 min run
milk shake, 10 oz	500	50 min jog or 25 min run
potato chips, 25	250	50 min of slow cycling or 1⅔ hr stroll
Big Mac	550	55 min of fast cycling or 55 min jog
pizza, 14"	2000	13⅓ hr stroll or 1⅔ hr run

*Note: The above table assumes the calories used per minute (based on a 150 lb male) to be:

Activity	Miles per Hour	Calories/Minute
stroll	1	2.5
brisk walk	4	7
slow jog	5	10
run	10	20
slow cycle	5	5
fast cycle	13	10

Remember that these are estimates only, used to illustrate caloric use in a comprehensible manner.

Do not let these facts fool or discourage you about the importance of exercise in controlling weight. The calorie-expending effects of exercise are cumulative. You may not want to spend 15 whole days just walking in order to lose 15 pounds, but twenty minutes of brisk walking every day over the course of a year can achieve the same result. Weight loss with exercise occurs during the course of time, be it hours or years.

The calories used in physical activity, like the calories provided by food, affect total caloric balance and thereby affect body weight. The following chart clearly illustrates how moderate daily exercise can contribute to weight loss. Note that these are only estimates, since a wide range of caloric values exists, depending on individual differences, intensities of participation, and environmental variances such as weather, temperature, and altitude. But theoretically, if one engaged in the given exercises while consuming one's exact caloric requirements, the listed weight losses could be achieved.

STEP 4: RELEARNING

Just as you learned how to walk when you were an infant, you can now learn how to exercise. All it takes is determination, patience, and the desire to improve your present lifestyle. Changes need not be dramatic. In a manner similar to that used in modifying your food intake patterns, you can gradually change your undesirable activity patterns. By taking a careful look at your present level of physical activity, you can then begin to gradually replace your sedentary habits with more active behaviors. The chart on the next page may assist you in doing so.

In Column A, list all physical activities regularly engaged in. (Select your activities from the Activity List on page 200 and add any others not listed.) All activities listed should be moderate or strenuous in intensity (see Day Nine).

In Column B, approximate the length of time you usually spend undertaking each activity.

In Column C, indicate about how often each activity is engaged in.

In Column D, total the approximate amount of time spent for each activity (B × C = D).

Finally, total the average amount of time spent each week engaged in physical activity. How many minutes do you exercise each week? One hour per week, preferably in three 20-minute segments, is considered to be a physically-fit exercise pattern. Did your total approximate this amount?

Type of Exercise	Hours of Preparation	No. Calories Used Per Minute	No. Pounds Lost in Time Span
basketball	2/day	5.0 to 11.0	5 to 11 in 1 month
cycling (8 to 13 mph)	2/day	5.0 to 11.0	60 to 132 in 1 year
dancing	3/wk	7.0	9 to 10 in 6 months
gardening	4/wk	4.0 to 8.0	14 to 28 in 1 year
golfing (carrying clubs)	4/wk	6.0	21 to 22 in 1 year
handball	2/wk	11.0	12 in 8 months
hiking (3 mph)	6/wk	7.0	8 to 9 in 3 months
jogging (5 to 7 mph)	7/wk	10.0 to 14.5	62 to 90 in 1 year
karate and judo	3/wk	11.7	20 in 6 months
rope skipping (rigorous)	3/wk	13.3	2 to 3 in 1 month
rowing (4 mph)	1/wk	8.3	6 in 6 months
running (10 mph)	7/wk	21.4	10 in 1 month
sailing	6/wk	5.0	6 in 3 months
skating (leisurely)	3/wk	7.0	18 to 20 in 1 year
skiing (rigorous)	7/wk	10.0	30 in 6 months
skiing, x-country (4 mph)	7/wk	10.0	15 in 3 months
squash	2/wk	11.0	6 in 4 months
swimming (leisurely)	2/day	6.0 to 8.3	70 to 105 in 1 year
swimming (fast crawl)	2/day	6.0 to 12.5	70 to 140 in 1 year
tennis	6/wk	6.0 to 8.0	32 to 42 in 1 year
volleyball	2/wk	5.0 to 7.5	1 to 2 in 3 months
walking (stroll)	7/wk	2.5	15 in 1 year
walking (3 to 4 mph)	7/wk	5.0 to 7.0	30 to 40 in 1 year

Note: Caloric consumption based on 154 pound person; there is a 10% increase in caloric consumption for each 15.4 pounds over this weight, and a 10% decrease for each 15.4 pounds under this weight.

Column A: Activity	Column B: Duration (in minutes)	Column C: No. Times Per Week	Column D: Total Time Per Activity

Total Time Per Week: _____ minutes

Activity List and Benefits

Activity	Heart*	Endurance	Strength	Flexibility	Coordination
Aerobic dancing	X	X	X	X	X
Basketball	X	X	X		X
Boxing	X	X		X	X
Canoeing	X	X	X		X
Climbing	X	X	X		
Cycling (9.4 mph or more)	X	X	X		
Dancing (except ballroom)	X				X
Fencing	X			X	X
Field hockey	X	X	X		X
Football	X	X	X		
Horseback riding	X	X	X		X
Ice hockey	X	X	X		X
Judo and karate	X	X	X	X	X
Handball	X	X	X	X	X
Racquetball	X	X	X	X	X
Rope skipping	X	X			
Running	X	X	X		
Sailing	X	X	X		X
Skiing	X	X			
Snow shoeing	X	X	X		
Soccer	X	X	X		X
Squash	X	X	X	X	X
Swimming	X	X	X		
Tennis	X	X	X	X	X
Volleyball	X				X
Walking, brisk	X	X			

*To significantly strengthen the cardiovascular system, the activity should be undertaken without rest for twenty minutes or more.

Remember that, among other benefits, regular physical exercise will provide you with the following:

- strengthened cardiovascular system
- improved muscle endurance
- increased muscle strength
- increased flexibility
- improved coordination

Note which of these important health benefits can be obtained from engaging in the various activities listed above. And most of these activities can prove to be really fun, too!

STEP 5: DAY-TO-DAY ACTIVITIES

The typical daily routine of the average American includes behaviors which serve to reduce the amount of time spent being physically active. By making some minor alterations in your present lifestyle, your day-to-day activity level can be modified so that you spend less time being sedentary, and more time in physical activity. The following suggestions can help you to change some of your sedentary behaviors to thereby increase your day-to-day activity level:

- Park your car or get off the bus several blocks away from your destination and walk the rest of the way—briskly.
- When traveling a short distance, ride a bicycle or walk.
- Use coffee breaks to exercise—take a brisk walk, stretch, do calisthenics.
- Use your lunch hour to exercise—take a brisk walk, jog, or play tennis.
- Arise half an hour earlier than usual to exercise —walk, jog, ride a bicycle.
- Use stairs instead of elevators.
- Involve yourself in active household duties such as sweeping, gardening, lawn mowing, painting, floor waxing, shoveling, etc.
- Get a dog and walk it daily.
- Be your own golf caddy.
- When bored, avoid the urge to eat and involve yourself in physical activity instead.

STEP 6: YOUR ACTIVITY PLAN

In addition to making day-to-day behavior modifications in your physical activities, you may want to use the activity plan on page 202 to create your own program of regular exercise. A sample activity plan is given to illustrate how to develop your own plan. In developing your activity plan, keep in mind the following suggestions:

1) Select physical activities which you enjoy and wish to incorporate into your activity plan. Include a variety of different activities to lessen the chances of boredom.

2) Set goals for:
- length of time spent each day per activity.
- distance covered or number of repetitions for each activity.

Do not push yourself too hard. Progress gradually to avoid overexertion and the possibility of developing distaste for the activities.

3) Set aside specific times during the day to engage in your chosen activities. Avoid excusing yourself from participation in activities; it is a lot easier to devise reasons not to exercise, than it is to get up and do it!

4) Exercise with others whenever possible. An exercise "buddy" can help prevent boredom and may assist you in adhering to your activity plan.

5) Reward yourself for meeting goals: buy yourself a new pair of sneakers or a tennis outfit, join an exclusive health club, or indulge yourself in a long, hot bath after exercising. Avoid using food as a reward, however; return to old undesirable eating habits should not accompany the development of new activity patterns.

STEP 7: PRE-ACTIVITY EATING

Meals should be eaten three to four hours prior to vigorous exercise to allow for complete digestion and to avoid stomach cramping. Foods to avoid before exercising include:

- fatty foods
- gas-forming foods
- caffeine-containing beverages
- alcoholic beverages
- salt tablets

Fatty foods are slow to digest, so may interfere with efficiency in exercise. Gas-forming foods can cause discomfort and thereby detract from physical ability. Caffeine and alcohol act as diuretics, and excess fluid losses can result in dehydration. Dehydration interferes with endurance and has led to death, notably in athletes and particularly in hot, humid environments. If physical activity is to continue for more than 15 minutes, lost fluids should be replaced. Note that thirst is not always a reliable indicator of rehydration needs. Special supplements are not required, however, to replace lost fluids. Nor are salt tablets required to replace the salt which is lost along with body fluids during exercise. Water is actually the fluid replacement of

---

Sample Activity Plan

1) Activities: *jogging, walking, tennis, health club "work-out"*

2) Goals—Long-term: *be able to jog 5 miles*
Immediate: *walk every day until progress to jogging, improve tennis game*

3) Activity Times:

Monday	Tuesday	Wednesday	Thursday	Friday	Saturday	Sunday
7 am walk/jog	——————————————————————————————————→				tennis AM	
	Health Club 7 to 8 pm		Health Club 7 to 8 pm			walk/jog PM

4) "Buddies": *walk/jog—husband Harry; tennis—sister Sue; health club—neighbor Nancy*

5) Rewards: *new sneakers when able to jog one mile; new tennis outfit after attending weekly match for four months straight; join the country club health club if attend local club as planned for next six months*

Activity Plan

1) Activities: _____
_____
_____

2) Goals—Long-Term: _____
        Immediate: _____
_____

3) Activity Times:

Monday	Tuesday	Wednesday	Thursday	Friday	Saturday	Sunday

4) "Buddies": _____
_____
_____

5) Rewards: _____
_____
_____
_____

---

choice, and the salt present in the average diet can usually meet increased needs. In especially hot weather, those involved in strenuous exercise may want to add a shake or two of salt to their meals to ensure replacement of sodium losses.

Special health foods, protein supplements, and vitamin-mineral preparations may serve to unbalance the diet, drain the bank account, and damage health. A well-balanced diet composed of a variety of foods in moderate amounts is usually sufficient to meet bodily needs, even during strenuous exercise programs.

Imagine that you are about to embark on a five-mile run at 3 PM; select (✓) the sample noontime meal from the choices below which would best enhance your performance:

____ a) Hamburger on bun, French fries, tossed salad with bleu cheese dressing, milk, apple

____ b) Super-shake—whole milk, ice cream, egg, honey, protein powder, wheat germ

____ c) T-bone steak, home fries, coleslaw, rolls and butter, cheesecake

____ d) Coffee and donuts

____ e) Beer and peanuts

____ f) Broiled chicken, brown rice, green beans, skim milk, baked apple

The best menu choice is f) because it is low in fat, non-gaseous, and does not contain either caffeine or alcohol. This luncheon is also well balanced, high in carbohydrate and fiber, and absent of Others Group foods...a wise selection for pre-activity, post-activity, or non-activity eating!

STEP 8: DAY TWENTY-FIVE PLAN

On Day Twenty-Five, continue to follow your weekly menu planner (see Day Twenty-Two). Try to include some of the smart snacks and recommended recipes from Days Twenty-One and Twenty-Three. At the end of Day Twenty-Five, use red ink to circle all planned foods which were not included and to write in any unplanned items you may have eaten. How closely did you approximate your menu planner for Day Twenty-Five? For what reasons did you deviate from your plan?

For the next five days, starting on Day Twenty-Five, list all of the physical activities you engage in. Each time you undertake a physical activity, record the date, time, and how long the activity was sustained; add any pertinent comments or feelings you may have concerning the activity itself and/or your own involvement. Keep in mind the following questions:

• Are you participating in the various activities included in your activity plan?

• Did you achieve any of your immediate goals?
• Did you avoid devising excuses to postpone planned physical activities?
• Did you seek and obtain assistance from a "buddy" or "buddies"?
• Were you able to reward yourself? If so, how?

Continue to follow your activity plan, filling in the chart below, and asking yourself the above questions on Days Twenty-Six through Twenty-Nine. Remember that a regular program of physical activity can serve to enhance both physical and psychological well-being. And exercise can be fun, as well as healthy!

Activity	Date and Time	Duration (in minutes)	Comments and Feelings

DAY TWENTY-SIX

NUTRITION AND THE MIND

STEP 1: YOU ARE WHAT YOU EAT

Each of us has inherited the potential for obtaining a specific level of physical and mental health. Whether or not we realize our own potential depends extensively on nutritional status. Individuals who follow nutritionally inadequate diets may not suffer from debilitating malnutrition, but they can exhibit many undesirable physical and mental side effects.

Carefully consider your own psychological outlook and emotional characteristics as you answer the following questions as honestly as possible:

Often	Sometimes	Never	
☐	☐	☐	Do you feel emotionally drained?
☐	☐	☐	Are you nervous and "up-tight"?
☐	☐	☐	Are you irritated by trivial matters?
☐	☐	☐	Do you feel physically tired and dragged out?
☐	☐	☐	Do you have trouble falling asleep?
☐	☐	☐	Do you find it difficult to concentrate for any length of time?
☐	☐	☐	Do you find that your memory is poor?
☐	☐	☐	Do you find it difficult to make even a simple decision?
☐	☐	☐	Do you become depressed for indefinable reasons?
☐	☐	☐	Have you lost interest in short- and long-range endeavors?

Many different factors contribute to making us who we are. Heredity and environment are especially influential in constructing our individual selves. It is difficult, perhaps impossible, to separate these various influences. But what we choose to do with what we are is up to each of us.

Nutrition is an important part of our environment, and an aspect over which we have a good degree of control. A nutritionally deficient diet can result in any or all of the following symptoms:

1) lack of endurance
2) nervousness
3) irritability
4) continual fatigue
5) insomnia
6) decreased attention span
7) memory impairment
8) indecision
9) depression
10) lack of motivation

Obviously, emotional difficulties can be due to or magnified by an inadequate diet. A well-balanced diet, which includes a variety of nutritious foods in the amounts required to meet your individual needs, can assist your emotional as well as your physical health.

STEP 2: FOOD AND MOOD—FACT OR TBP?

During the past several decades, scientific research has unveiled a vast array of interrelationships between diet and physical disease. New research is now underway to determine the psychological effects of various dietary constituents. Most of this research is highly theoretical in nature, and few studies have yet resulted in documented evidence. Many of the proposed theories have been grasped by the scientifically untrained, blown out of proportion, and presented to the public as fact.

Some of the possible relationships between food intake and emotional moods are worth considering, and will soon be more completely researched. Until substantiated evidence disproves or supports these theories, however, it is important to weigh the facts before making your own decisions. Indicate whether you think the following theories are fact or TBP (to be proven).

Fact	TBP	
☐	☐	Food additives cause children to be hyperactive.
☐	☐	The B-vitamin niacin is an effective treatment for schizophrenia.

Fact	TBP	
☐	☐	Foods rich in tryptophan, a protein constituent related to nerve function, are sleep-inducing and may relieve depression.
☐	☐	Foods high in tyrosine, another protein constituent, may also relieve depression.
☐	☐	Use of choline, a vitamin derivative, may help to enhance memory.

All five of the above theories are currently under scientific investigation and each has yet TBP (to be proven). A brief survey of the information available on each of these theories reveals the following facts:

1) The Feingold Diet was developed by an allergist, the late Dr. Benjamin Feingold, of the Kaiser-Permanente Medical Center in Oakland, CA. Dr. Feingold's theory claims that hyperactive behavior in children is caused by an allergy to the following dietary constituents:

- artificial (synthetic) food colorings
- artificial (synthetic) food flavorings
- food additives BHA and BHT, commonly used as preservatives in dry cereals, salad dressings, vegetable oils and margarine.
- salicylate, a chemical compound found in pain medications such as aspirin, and naturally present in certain foods including cucumbers, tomatoes, apples, apricots, cherries, grapes, nectarines, oranges, peaches, plums, prunes, raisins, raspberries, strawberries, and tea.

Researchers have estimated that 5% to 10% of all American children can be classified as "hyperactive," as defined by repeated display of the following symptoms:

- short attention span
- excessive purposeless activity
- irrational behavior
- destructiveness and hostility
- insomnia

Since the publication of Feingold's popular book, *Why Your Child is Hyperactive*, thousands of so-called hyperactive children have adopted his suggested diet. The "Feingold Diet," which eliminates all foods containing artificial colorings, artificial flavorings, salicylates, and most recently BHT and BHA, is as difficult for most parents to administer as it is impractical for most children to adhere to. Most foods (including breads) must be prepared at home from scratch, restaurant and school meals are usually not allowed, and all food intake must be carefully monitored. In excluding many commonly available foods, including various fruits and vegetables, special care must be taken to ensure that the diet is nutritionally balanced.

Despite the multitude of success stories from convinced parents, scientifically conducted studies have repeatedly failed to support the theory. Alternative dietary factors—including caffeine—have been suggested as causes for hyperactive behavior in children, and further study needs to be conducted. At the present time, most nutritionists and doctors believe that it is probably a combination of several factors which cause any behavioral improvements associated with the Feingold Diet, including the following:

- The diet is well balanced, which may result in improved nutritional status and enhance overall physical and mental health.
- Elimination of caffeine could calm the nervous system and affect blood sugar levels, influencing behavior and mood.
- Instituting the diet is usually a family effort, which draws the family together and provides the child with extra support.
- By providing a tangible cause for the child's behavioral problems, the diet can alleviate parental guilt so that they are able to cope with the situation more rationally.
- By providing the child with a sense of responsibility, the diet can assist the child to adopt more mature attitudes and behaviors.

Most health professionals do not advocate the Feingold Diet because there exists no scientific evidence to substantiate its use and it creates a false dependence on diet for determining behaviors. However, a well-balanced diet in a supportive family environment is certainly a desirable alternative to hyperactivity and the frustrations and mental anguish it entails.

2) Niacin, one of the B-vitamins, assists in the proper function of the nervous system, and a deficiency can result in such nervous disorders as depression, insomnia, and mental confusion. Due to the role of niacin in the overall health of the nervous system, experimental treatment of schizophrenics using very large doses of this vitamin were initiated. Results, however, have been dissatisfying, and the side effects associated with large intakes of niacin are both irritating and dangerous. A true niacin deficiency will respond to vitamin supplementation, but scientific evidence does not support the concept that schizophrenics are niacin deficient. Further research in the area of diet and depression, however, warrants support. A well-balanced diet with accompanying improvements in physical health could serve to enhance the emotional status of anyone undergoing psychological difficulties, including the schizophrenic.

3) An injection or oral dosage of pure tryptophan will elevate brain levels of serotonin, a

chemical important in nerve function. Neither tryptophan nor serotonin, however, have been shown to be elevated in the brain when protein foods rich in tryptophan are eaten. Following further research, however, dietary adjustments may eventually be used in conjunction with prescribed doses of tryptophan to treat insomnia and depression. Study in this area is just beginning, and careful consideration should be given to any advertisement of diets or nutritional supports which claim to improve mental disorders.

4) As with tryptophan, dietary adjustments may eventually be used in conjunction with prescribed doses of tyrosine as part of the treatment of depression. A diet containing large amounts of foods high in tyrosine, however, is currently believed to prevent the elevation of brain levels of tyrosine. Further research is underway, and again, advertised claims which advocate dietary treatment of psychological disorders are usually undocumented.

5) Dietary increases in choline are reflected as blood elevations of choline. Investigation is currently underway to determine the beneficial effects, if any, of the subsequent stimulation of certain nervous system components. Most commercially sold choline preparations (labeled as "choline" or "lecithin") do not provide the proper amount of choline required to affect the nervous system. Research in the area of nutrition and memory is as exciting in its possibilities as it is absent in its conclusions so far.

Study on all five of the above theories is relatively new, and a good deal more research will have to be completed before we have a clear view of food-mood interrelationships. Until such a time, however, be conscious of how certain foods affect your moods: individuals are all uniquely affected by what and how much they eat. Have you noticed any improvement in mental outlook, lessened sleeping difficulties, and/or enhanced self-confidence since you began modifying your diet and working to better your health and well-being?

STEP 3: MORE FACTS ON FOOD AND MOOD

Approximately 25% of our population suffers from allergies, some of which are related to specific foods. The foods which are most commonly accused of causing allergic responses include:

- milk
- eggs
- wheat
- chocolate
- nuts
- fish and shellfish
- berries
- peas
- citrus fruits
- corn

Allergy testing is long and involved, and includes clinical diagnosis procedures, laboratory testing, and elimination diets (in which almost all foods are restricted, then gradually added back to the diet, in order to try to isolate the allergy-inducers). Even with all the expensive testing, results may not be definitive. Thus, we need to be wary of claims which state that behavioral disorders are merely allergic reactions to foods (see Step 2), simple to identify and treat. In most cases, mental dysfunctions are due to causes far more complex than food reactions.

We should also be careful to evaluate any claims for the use of vitamin supplements or so-called health foods in the treatment of emotional disturbances. Psychological problems are highly intricate, and it is extremely difficult to determine the causes. Use of dietary constituents usually has only a placebo effect, if any, and does not assist in delineating the reasons for such disorders. Most diet claims are ineffective, and merely serve as a temporary way to avoid facing complex, deep-seated emotional needs.

However, food can play an important role in helping to determine mental health, as well as overall physical status. A nutritionally inadequate diet leads to observable signs of physical and psychological imbalance:

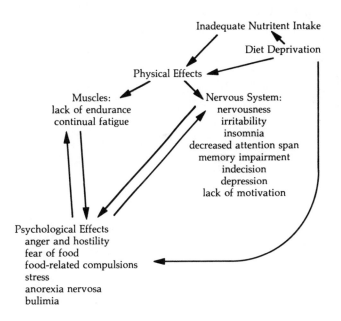

Inadequate Nutrient Intake

Diet Deprivation

Physical Effects

Muscles:
lack of endurance
continual fatigue

Nervous System:
nervousness
irritability
insomnia
decreased attention span
memory impairment
indecision
depression
lack of motivation

Psychological Effects
anger and hostility
fear of food
food-related compulsions
stress
anorexia nervosa
bulimia

Obviously, diet has a direct effect on both physical and psychological status. A well-balanced diet that includes a variety of nutritious foods can help to support a fit body and a healthy mind.

Note: If you are having serious psychological problems, be they diet-related or otherwise, it is important that you consult your physician and/or professional counselor. Diet alone is probably not the answer, and reliance on special foods or supplements can delay needed help.

STEP 4: DAY TWENTY-SIX PLAN

On Day Twenty-Six, continue to follow your weekly menu planner (see Day Twenty-Two). Try to include some of the smart snacks and recommended recipes from Days Twenty-One and Twenty-Three. At the end of Day Twenty-Six, use red ink to circle all planned foods which were not included and to write in any unplanned items you may have eaten. How closely did you approximate your menu planner for Day Twenty-Six? For what reasons did you deviate from your plan?

Continue to record all of your physical activities (see Step 8, Day Twenty-Five). A well-balanced diet and a program of regular physical exercise can help to improve your psychological, as well as physical, well-being. And reduction in mental stresses can assist you to adhere to both your Nutri-Plan diet plan and your activity plan.

Are you stressed? Did you find yourself answering Often or Sometimes to most of the questions in Step 1? If so, stress reduction techniques may be of vital assistance in alleviating your emotional tensions and the associated physical and mental disturbances. There are several different stress reduction programs currently available to the public, including:

- Transcendental Meditation (TM)
- Yoga
- Hypnosis
- Exercises-for-relaxation courses
- Stress-relaxation courses

Your emotional environment, like your diet, needs to be well-balanced so that you can maintain an optimal level of both physical and psychological well-being. Call it: "feeling good all over!"

DAY TWENTY-SEVEN

HOW ABOUT HEALTH FOODS?

STEP 1: DEFINING "HEALTH FOOD"

During the past decade, there has been a considerable upsurge in public interest in the relationship of diet and health: consumers want to know which foods to eat in order to promote good health, and which foods to avoid in order to delay the onset of disease and old age. There has also been a simultaneous increase in the spread of nutrition misinformation and health quackery. There exist a multitude of claims for specific foods that proposedly prevent or cure disease and old age, or that provide other special health benefits. Bookshelves are bulging with paperbacks promoting anti-arthritis vitamins, anti-cancer diets, anti-depression foods, anti-aging regimens, and anti-fat miracle cures. It is difficult for the average consumer to separate fact from fad.

In your own words, define the following terms:

1) "natural food" _____
_____
_____

2) "organic food" _____
_____
_____

3) "health food" _____
_____
_____

These three terms have no legal definition, and are often used interchangeably. Usually they mean whatever the manufacturer of the product so-labeled wants them to mean. One of the most popular areas of nutrition misconception centers around the use and abuse of these three terms.

These three terms indicate a variety of possibilities about a product to consumers. A product labeled "natural" or "organic" is usually thought of as a "health food" and assumed to:

- contain no artificial coloring or flavorings
- contain no additives or artificial preservatives
- be unrefined and unprocessed
- be grown without use of synthetic fertilizers or pesticides
- be health-giving and "good for you"
- be a superfood

The so-called health foods do not necessarily promote good health. In fact, health food stores often promote the following foods that have caloric contents which outweigh nutrient values:

- brown sugar, "raw" sugar, fructose
- potato chips, corn chips, other salty snack foods
- ice cream with high fat contents
- cookies, cakes, other sweets
- candy

A careful look at the labels for these products will reveal that they may differ from their supermarket counterparts in that they supposedly are free of additives, preservatives, and/or refined sugar. However, the informed shopper is aware of the following facts:

- Brown sugar, "raw" sugar, and fructose are all highly refined, contribute little to the diet besides calories, and are an unnecessarily expensive way to sweeten the diet; table sugar is nutritionally equivalent and significantly less expensive.

- Chips and other salty snack foods are high in fat-calories, and the sea salt added to many health foods is as undesirably rich in sodium as table salt.

- "Natural" ice creams tend to contain more calories—more butter fat and lots of honey—while costs are prohibitive.

- Dessert-type foods sold as health foods are merely costly alternatives to homemade, bakery, or store-bought items; the absence of additives and the addition of honey does little to alter the high-calorie, low-nutrient values of such products.

- Even though they may sound healthy—"Health

Bar," "Power Crunch," "Fitness Chews"—the labels prove that the main difference between such products and regular candy is the cost.

The increased marketability of foods labeled as "natural" has had noticeable impact on the food industry. Supermarkets currently offer a wide variety of "natural" products, including cereals, juices, chips, ice cream, candy bars, peanut butter, even beer. Aware consumers may ask themselves what is so natural about deep-fat fried, highly-salted corn chips, and what is the difference between fruit juices labeled as natural and those that are not. Perhaps the answers will become clear when the prices are compared to those of various "unnatural" products. It seems that almost every level of the food industry spectrum, from the individual health food market to the international food manufacturer, is currently taking advantage of both legally undefined labeling terminology and the nutrition naiveté of consumers.

The US government is presently undertaking legal action to define these three popular and confusing terms. Until "health food," "organic," and "natural" have legal definitions, however, it is up to you, as an informed consumer, to make the wisest food shopping decisions possible. Your health status and food budget will thank you for it.

STEP 2: FACT OR FAD?

Quackery is a term derived from the word "quicksilver," which means "to boast of a cure." Back in the good old days, quacks promoted patent medicines and revitalizing tonics. Today, quacks still try to sell us their health-giving miracle products. Nutritional charlatans have always been able to peddle their wares because of the widespread existence of health misconceptions. In order to avoid falling prey to health charlatans, and to be able to evaluate the food industry's advertising claims, consumers simply need to transform their nutrition misconceptions into nutrition knowledge.

You may want to begin to clear up your own nutrition fallacies by selecting either Fact or Fad to describe each of the following statements:

Fact Fad
☐ ☐ The American food supply is devitalized and can no longer maintain our good health.

☐ ☐ Natural vitamin and mineral preparations are nutritionally superior to synthetic supplements.

☐ ☐ Foods that are grown in organically fertilized soils are far more nutritious than products grown in chemically fertilized soils.

The nutritional deficiency diseases, which were once major health problems in this country, have nearly disappeared. (These deficiencies can still occur, however, with alcoholism, poverty, ignorance, and food faddism.) The American food supply now offers us a wider variety of nutritious foods than at any other time in history: we can have vitamin C-rich mangoes from Florida, potassium-rich bananas from the tropics, iodized salt, nutrient-enriched breads and cereals, and many kinds of food products from all over the world nearly anytime we desire. Our foods are available in many different forms—fresh, frozen, canned, and dried, boxed, bottled, bagged, and bare. With careful selection and nutrition know-how, we can readily select a well-balanced, healthy diet from the current American food supply.

Neither the body nor plants can distinguish between naturally occurring chemicals and man-made chemicals. There is no nutritional difference between natural and synthetic vitamins, and the nutritional value of "organically" grown foods is equivalent to that of foods grown in chemically fertilized soil. The only significant difference lies in the price: organic foods and natural vitamins often cost far more than their non-health food counterparts.

Fact Fad
☐ ☐ Ginseng can cause high blood pressure, and other herbs have been known to prove dangerous, even fatal.

Ginseng, a popular herbal remedy touted as a cure for a variety of disorders ranging from impotence to fatigue, has been shown to contribute to high blood pressure. Ginseng can also irritate the gastric and nervous systems, causing diarrhea, nervousness, and insomnia.

Pennyroyal oil, used in teas since the Roman days to regulate menstruation and to induce abortion, recently resulted in death: an eighteen-year-old women died after consuming only one ounce of the herb, and the autopsy uncovered kidney and liver damage.

Sassafras bark tea can also prove dangerous. The primary ingredient is safrole, a known cancer-causing agent in animals. The Food and Drug Administration recently banned the use of this herb as a flavoring agent, but the tea is still popular.

Just because a food or beverage is derived from leaves or roots does not guarantee safety. Susceptible individuals may experience adverse reactions to normal amounts of naturally occurring dietary constituents, while excessively large amounts can prove fatal (more on this topic on Day Twenty-Eight).

The following herbs are of questionable safety and use is not recommended:

- ginseng
- pennyroyal
- sassafras
- licorice root (increased blood pressure)
- poke root, senna root, dock roots, aloe (diarrhea, vomiting)
- burdock root (hallucinations)
- chamomile, goldenrod, marigold, yarrow (severe allergic reactions in those sensitive to ragweed and related plants)
- St-John's-wort (sun sensitivity)
- catnip, juniper, hydrangea, jimson weed, lobelia, nutmeg, wormwood (nervous system poisoning)
- alfalfa (disrupted digestion and respiration)
- comfrey (liver and bladder tumors in laboratory animals)

Fact Fad
☐   ☐   Bee pollen is rich in nutrients, and is an especially good source of vitamin B_{15}.

Remember that vitamins are essential substances which we must obtain through our diets in the amounts required for normal growth and proper body function. Legitimate vitamins have been proven as essential for adequate human nutrition. "Vitamin" B_{15} has not been demonstrated as essential for human growth and function, and actually is not even a vitamin. Products labeled as B_{15} may contain a variety of different substances, including a stimulant with possibly harmful side effects. Nor have any nutritional benefits been established for bee pollen. The false promotion of substances as vitamins or as health-promoting aids are usually merely money-making schemes. The nutritionally educated consumer can evaluate such claims, and thereby avoid possible health damage and unnecessary money expenditure.

Fact Fad
☐   ☐   Wheat germ, brewer's yeast, and protein powder are superfoods with special health promoting ingredients.

Wheat germ and brewer's yeast can provide a significant amount of several vitamins and minerals, while protein powders are either composed of dried milk, or of synthetic amino acids (protein components) which are often inadequate in protein quality. A well-balanced diet makes such supplementary food products unnecessary, and high prices often make them undesirable. There are no superfoods, and all foods promote good health when part of a nutritionally complete diet.

Obviously, a combination of common sense and nutritional know-how can protect your health and lower your food bills. As always, the choice and responsibility are up to you.

STEP 3: CHARTING YOUR WAY

How can you identify health food frauds, health quackery and nutrition mythology? Every time you encounter health food claims, "natural" labels, or disease-curing diet plans, ask yourself the following questions:

1) Is the product/book/person promising something that seems too good to be true? Is supernutrition offered as a cure for the incurable, or as a means to prevent the inevitable?

2) Does the product/book/person rely on testimonials and case histories rather than on scientific data in order to support any claims?

3) Has the product/book/person been reviewed by qualified experts with recognized nutrition degrees from reputable universities?

4) Will the product/book/person promote the concept that diet alone can prevent and cure disease? This is an especially dangerous concept which can lead to economically and nutritionally unfavorable consequences, and may result in illness and death.

Health food mythology is a serious business, one the consumer needs to be adept at evaluating. You may want to use the chart on pages 212–213 in order to identify some popular health foods, the associated nutritional claims, and their scientifically factual qualities.

STEP 4: DAY TWENTY-SEVEN PLAN

On Day Twenty-Seven, continue to follow your weekly menu planner from Day Twenty-Two and continue to record all of your physical activities in the chart from Day Twenty-Five. Also, try to keep emotional stress to a minimum. Involve yourself in a commercial or self-designed stress reduction program, and make sure that your emotional environment, like your diet, is well balanced.

For Day Twenty-Seven, do some comparative shopping. On the chart on page 213, list six products in your kitchen that are labeled as "health foods," "natural," or "organic." List each price and any nutritional claims. (If necessary, visit a nearby health food store and your local supermarket to add enough products to the list in order to total six.) At the supermarket, find six foods comparable to the listed health foods, and list these items and their prices. Total the costs for the health food buys and the comparable "unnatural" items. How much money could you have saved by avoiding the purchase of health food items? Are any of the nutritional claims associated with these health food items substantiated by scientific evidence? Compare each listed health food with the chart given in Step 3. Do any of these items have associated nutritional myths? Do any of your listed health foods pose possible health dangers? Are they worth the cost... to both your health and your budget?

What's so healthy about "health foods?" Any nutritious food, eaten in proper amounts, supports health. There are no "magic" foods with special health-giving properties, and an excess of (*) items has been shown to be dangerous to health.

"Health Food"	Claim(s)	Scientific Fact(s)
Acerola cherry	Excellent source of vitamin C	Citrus fruits more readily available
Acidophilus	Helps restore normal intestinal flora	Intestinal flora function well in normal healthy people
Alfalfa	Has minerals lacking in shallow-root plants	Subsoils have fewer nutrients than topsoils
Almonds	Excellent source of calcium	Calcium equivalent to one cup milk, with thrice the calories
Bee pollen	Rich in nourishing factors and enzymes	No special nutrients; mostly fruit sugar
Biotin	Prevents baldness and restores hair	No known deficiency in humans; no proven effects on hair growth
Blackstrap molasses	Enriches blood, provides energy	High in iron and sugar
Bone meal*	Halts muscle pain, menstrual cramps, nervous problems	Good source calcium, but may contain toxic metals
Bran*	Prevents appendicitis and cancer of the colon	Increases bulk, aids digestion and elimination; excess can cause diarrhea, nutrient losses, intestinal blockage
Brewer's yeast	Lifts depression, restores genes	High in protein, B-complex vitamins
Brown rice	Adequate alone to maintain life	More nutrients than white rice but protein incomplete
Carob	Unrefined, nutritious chocolate substitute	Dried powder of seed pod (contains no caffeine); often added to high-fat, high-sugar foods
Choline	Enhances memory	No known deficiency in man; body makes own supply
Cider vinegar	Balances body's acid-ash content; cures kidney disease and overweight	Contains potassium which is widely distributed in foods
"Coaches' formula"*	Rebuilds muscle tissue; easily digested	Contains skim milk powder, sugar, enzymes; amino acid content may be unbalanced
Cod liver oil*	Excellent source vitamin D	Upsets proper digestion and nutrient absorption
Desiccated liver*	Aids body to make vitamin B_{12}	May conceal anemia; contains only some of the nutrients in liver
Dolomite*	Cures nerve and muscle disorders	Good source calcium, but may contain toxic metals
Enzymes	Aid digestion, decrease gas	Broken down during digestion; body makes own supply
Fertilized eggs	Better amino acid content	Equal nutritionally to unfertilized eggs
Garlic	Cures hypertension, cancer, skin disease; halts aging	Odor is absorbed into blood, breathed out through lungs; health benefits unproven
Ginseng*	Increases energy	Non-caloric herb; may elevate blood pressure
Glutamic acid	Inhibits gene breakdown, aids memory	Broken down during digestion; body makes own supply
Goat's milk	Highly nutritious and disease-free	No more nutritious than cow's milk; dangerous if unpasteurized
Granola	High in nutrients and fiber	High in calories, sugar, and fat
Honey	Cures arthritis, high in nutrients, useful for diabetics	Nutritionally similar to table sugar
Inositol	Clears blood of fat and cholesterol	No known deficiency in man; widely distributed in food
Kelp*	Natural source of iodine, other minerals	High in sodium
Lecithin	Dissolves cholesterol and clears blood of fat	Phospholipid in all cells; body makes own supply

"Health Food"	Claim(s)	Scientific Fact(s)
Minerals*	Cure variety of health problems and diseases	Widely distributed in food; deficiencies unknown or rare; can build up in body to toxic levels
"Organic" food	More nutritious than supermarket foods	No more nutritious; usually more expensive
Pantothenic acid	Calms anxiety, speeds healing, combats cancer	Deficiency unknown in man; widely distributed in food
Papain	Aids digestion, decreases gas	Broken down during digestion and deactified
Protein powders*	Builds muscle tissue	Nutritionally similar to skim milk powder; amino acid content may be unbalanced
Raw cheese*	More nutritious than pasteurized cheese	Dangerous if aged less than 60 days
Raw egg*	More nutrients, easily digested	Nutritionally equivalent to cooked eggs; chance of food poisoning from bacterial contamination
Raw meat*	More nutritious than cooked meat	Nutritionally equivalent to cooked; danger of toxoplasmosis, tapeworm, other diseases
Raw milk*	More nutritious than pasteurized milk	Nutritionally equivalent to pasteurized; danger of undulant fever, TB, other diseases
Raw nuts*	More nutritious than roasted nuts	Nutritionally equivalent to cooked; danger of aflatoxin infection
Raw sugar	Unrefined, with high nutrient content	Refined, with trace amounts of molasses on crystals
Rutin	Aids in complete utilization of vitamin C	Accompanies vitamin C in food sources
RNA/DNA	Inhibits gene breakdown, halts aging	Broken down during digestion; body makes own supply
Sea salt*	Unrefined; source of iodine, other minerals	Refined; high in sodium
Seeds	Excellent source of protein and energy	Incomplete protein; high in calories
"Tiger's milk"	High in protein, vitamins, energy	Contains skim milk powder, sugar, calories
Vitamins*	Inadequate in food supply, prevent and cure a variety of ills	Sufficiently available in food supply; excesses can cause side effects, sometimes toxic
Wheat germ	Nutritious, low-calorie, high energy supplement	Good source protein, vitamins; relatively high in calories, fat

*An excessive intake has been shown to be dangerous to health.

Health Food	Cost and Package Size	Nutritional Claims
1) 2) 3) 4) 5) 6)		

Total Cost: _____

Comparable Food	Cost and Package Size	Nutritional Claims, if any
1) 2) 3) 4) 5) 6)		

Total Cost: _____

DAY TWENTY-EIGHT

BAD TO ADD ADDITIVES?

STEP 1: AVOID ADDITIVES?

Indicate whether you think the following statement is True or False:

True False
□ □   Food additives are dangerous to our health.

There are over 2000 different substances currently being used as food additives. Most of these come from natural sources, or are identical or closely related to naturally occurring chemical components in foods. The typical American diet can be broken down by weight as follows:

- 99%—naturally occurring food components
- 1%—food additives
- trace amounts—pesticide residues, contaminants

Thus, it is those substances naturally present in foods which contribute to the diet the widest variety and largest amount of chemical substances.

Although many health dangers have been attributed to foodstuffs (eg, food poisonings, food allergies, nutritional diseases), no such hazard has ever been directly associated with food additives used according to government regulations. Additives are required to meet standard specifications of indentity and purity. The fact that a certain additive has an extended history of widespread dietary intake without harmful effects does not constitute acceptable proof of safety. In fact, the Food and Drug Administration is currently involved in the evaluation of those substances known as GRAS (generally recognized as safe), as well as all new food additives and certain other questionable additives.

Testing includes the feeding of each additive to at least two different animal species. In order to determine any cancer-causing possibilities, large doses are used; large amounts of most chemicals do not cause cancer, but if a large amount does, then usually a smaller dose will also—but with less frequency. There is always the chance that an additive will be of greater harm to humans than it is to animals. The reverse is also possible.

Due to a legal decision established in 1958 and known as the Delaney Clause, intentional food additives that may cause cancer in humans are not allowed to be used in any amount. This means that whenever laboratory testing implicates an additive as cancer-causing in animals, use of the additive is banned. However, naturally occurring food constituents that are known to induce cancer in humans or animals are not subject to this ruling. This is fortunate, as otherwise we would have an extremely limited choice of foods that we would be allowed to eat. Some common foods which contain naturally occurring cancer-causing chemicals include:

- beets (nitrates)
- lettuce (nitrates)
- radishes (nitrates)
- spinach (nitrates)
- olives (benzopyrene, tannins)
- sesame seed oil (sesamole)
- vegetable oils (benzopyrene)
- peanuts (aflatoxin molds)
- coffee (benzopyrene, caffeine, tannins)
- sassafras tea (safrole)
- tarragon (estragole)
- seaweed (carrageenan)

There exist in nature numerous other examples. Yet, the only food additive that has not been removed from the market after being classified as a potential cancer-causing agent is the artificial sweetener saccharin. Due to the voluminous public outcry over the possibility of a ban and the clamor made by the medical community as to the unreliability of the condemning studies, a temporary ruling was issued instead. This requires all products in interstate commerce containing saccharin to display the following warning label:

> "Use of this product may be hazardous to your health. This product contains saccharin which has been determined to cause cancer in laboratory animals."

Warning notices are also on display at all retail stores selling products which contain saccharin. Thus, the decision whether or not to use this sweetener is left up to us, as is the choice to consume sugar, salt, fatty foods, alcohol, and food itself. It is your responsibility to be an educated consumer so that you can make wise food selections. Perhaps an amendment in the Delaney Clause and a diminished tendency for over-regulation by our government will occur in the future. This could prove to be beneficial, however, only if accompanied by adequate consumer education.

STEP 2: AVOID FOOD ALTOGETHER?

Indicate whether you think the following question is True or False:

True False
☐ ☐ Foods are dangerous to our health.

Many substances are considered safe when consumed as a natural component of foods, but would not be acceptable as food additives. In fact, if all of the naturally occurring chemical components in foods were subject to the same safety evaluations required for food additives, many of us might starve!

If we were to apply the standards set by the US government for the determination of the safety of food additives, which of the additive-free foods from the menu below do you think would be banned:

olives   cheese chunks   carrot curls
           boiled shrimp with lemon
parslied potatoes   steamed broccoli
           fresh orange, apple, banana slices
milk   coffee   white wine

Each of the foods listed in the above menu contains chemical compounds which can be toxic in specific amounts. For example, carrots contain carrototoxin, a nerve poison. Lemon and parsley contain psoralen, a sunlight sensitizing agent. Shrimp contains arsenic. And vegetable oils, olives, smoked ham, and coffee all contain benzopyrene, a potent cancer-causing agent.

Actually, almost every food can be detrimental to health, either by being inherently poisonous (such as certain mushrooms), due to naturally occurring toxicants (as given in the above menu), or because of individual hypersensitivities or allergies. Despite the presence of such potential dangers in our food supply, we have managed to survive. It is obvious that the amounts of these naturally occurring chemicals are not sufficient to cause any direct harm.

This same principle can be applied to food additives. Consumed in moderate amounts by normal, healthy individuals, foods (composed of naturally occurring chemicals, with or without added chemical additives) are not dangerous to health. In fact, all foods contribute to good health when consumed in moderate amounts as part of a well-balanced and varied diet. However, most foods (with or without additives) can prove harmful if consumed in excessive amounts and/or eaten by susceptible individuals. Too much of anything, including too much of a good thing, can be toxic. Even water is unsafe in excessive amounts! Moderation is the wisest choice.

Bacterial contamination of food also poses a serious health hazard that affects more than 20 million Americans every year. Improper food handling, during processing or in the home, can lead to bacterial growth and result in food-borne illnesses. The flu-like symptoms are misdiagnosed by many afflicted individuals, and labeled as the "24-hour bug."

Thus, unlike unsanitary food, inadequate food supplies, or poor nutrition, a normal intake of food additives poses a negligible health risk. In fact, food additives can serve to increase the safety and nutritional value of our food supply.

Fortunately, we need not eliminate food—with naturally occurring chemicals and/or chemical additives—from our diets!

STEP 3: THE "GOOD" ONES?

The benefits of food additives for consumers are numerous, including the following:

• increased nutritional value of foods and overall diet
• varied food supply
• year-round food availability
• enhanced keeping quality
• decreased food costs

If the use of food additives were banned, surplus food stocks would quickly be depleted, baked goods would grow moldy and stale overnight, salad dressings and oils would separate and turn rancid, beverages would taste flat, and insects would infest cereals and grains. The many benefits for health and economic welfare certainly serve to justify the small degree of theoretical risk associated with the use of food additives. Each of the 2000 or so food additives approved for use is utilized in order to achieve a specific effect. In evaluating the usefulness of a particular food additive, the following factors should be considered:

• the advantages of using the additive.

- the consequences of not using the additive.
- any possible risks associated with both short- and long-term usage.

As always, the choice is yours: it is up to you to determine the degree of risk—minimal at most—you are willing to take in order to enjoy a varied, nutritious diet containing affordable foods that keep well and are available all year long. You may want to use the chart below for assistance in the identification of some common food additives. Note that asterisks (*) indicate those items currently under study due to inconclusive research indicating possible health risks. Research so far, however, has not demonstrated that serious harm from normal intakes is at all likely. In fact, most of our sodium nitrate intake comes from the amounts naturally present in many vegetables; nitrite is present in significant amounts in saliva, while both BHA and BHT may actually help to prevent certain cancers. The EDTA added to beer, carbonated drinks, salad dressings, mayonnaise, and certain sauces may bind up iron, making excessively large intakes inadvisable for anyone with a diagnosed iron deficiency.

STEP 4: THE "BAD" ONES?

Food additives help to ensure the large number and variety of products required to feed our large and varied populace. Additives serve to maintain or improve nutritional value, and they help to retain freshness in foods.

Food additives are also used to enhance product sales by assisting in food processing and increasing market appeal. This type of additive is used only to cater to our current love of convenience and our aesthetic desires. These additives are more widely used and more controversial, yet less important since they are added to foods to improve taste and appearance, not to enhance safety or nutritional value. In fact, the *most* common food additives are sugar and salt! You are already aware of the various nutritional consequences associated with an immoderate intake of either of these two products (see Day Fifteen).

Again, in evaluating the usefulness of a particular additive, the following factors should be considered:

- the advantages of using the additive.
- the consequences of not using the additive.
- any possible risks associated with both short- and long-term usage.

As always, the choice is yours: it is up to you to determine the degree of risk—minimal at most—you are willing to take, in order to enjoy a varied, nutritious diet containing foods which are convenient and aesthetically appealing. You may want to

Maintain or Improve Quality

Nutrients - enrich (replace vitamins and/or minerals removed in processing) or fortify (add nutrients which may be low in typical diet)	Preservatives - prevent spoilage, extend shelf life, or protect natural odor and/or flavor	Anti-oxidants - prevent or delay rancidity or enzyme-caused browning
Ascorbic acid (vitamin C)	Ascorbic acid (vitamin C)	Ascorbic acid (vitamin C)
Beta carotene (vitamin A)	Benzoic acid	BHA (butylated hydroxyanisole)*
Iodine	Butylparaben	BHT (butylated hydroxytoluene)*
Iron	Calcium lactate	Citric acid
Niacinamide	Calcium propionate	EDTA (ethylenediamine tetra-acetic acid)*
Potassium Iodide	Citric acid	Propyl gallate
Riboflavin	Heptylparaben	TBHQ (tertiary butylhydroquinone)
Thiamin	Lactic acid	Tocopherols (vitamin E)
Tocopherols (vitamin E)	Methyl paraben	
Vitamin D	Potassium propionate	
	Potassium sorbate	
	Propionic acid	
	Propylparaben	
	Sodium benzoate	
	Sodium diacetate	
	Sodium erythorbate	
	Sodium nitrate*	
	Sodium nitrite*	
	Sodium propionate	
	Sodium sorbate	
	Sorbic acid	

use the chart below for assistance in the identification of some common food additives. Note that asterisks (*) indicate those items currently under study due to inconclusive research indicating possible health risks. Research so far, however, has not demonstrated that serious harm from normal intake is at all likely. In fact, this type of additive is certainly not to be considered "bad," but necessary for self-indulgence and dining pleasure.

STEP 5: DAY TWENTY-EIGHT PLAN

On Day Twenty-Eight, continue to follow your weekly menu planner from Day Twenty-Two and to record all of your physical activities in the chart from Day Twenty-Five. Try to keep emotional stress to a minimum, and make sure that your emotional environment—like your diet—is well-balanced. Utilize your nutrition know-how in evaluating the use of health foods in your diet. Are they worth the price—considering your health and your budget?

For Day Twenty-Eight, consider the following concepts:

- Food additives comprise less than 99% of the total weight of the typical diet.
- Food additives are thoroughly tested by the Food and Drug Administration prior to use, and testing is continued, even after acceptance.
- If we applied the governmental standards for acceptance to the natural chemical components of all foodstuffs, most of our common foods and beverages would be outlawed.
- Most naturally occurring and chemically derived food components are not dangerous to health when eaten in moderate amounts by normal individuals.
- Certain additives (nutrients, preservatives, antioxidants) help to ensure us of a diet which contains a variety of nutritious foods at reasonable prices and with practical shelf lives.
- Certain additives (flavor enhancers, flavors, colors, sweeteners, emulsifiers, stabilizers, tex-

Affect Food Appeal

Flavor Enhancers - change or increase original taste and/or aroma without donating own taste	Flavors - increase or restore flavors	Colors - add desirable or characteristic color	Sweeteners - change or increase sweetness of taste and/or aroma
disodium guanylate disodium inosinate hydrolyzed vegetable protein MSG (monosodium glutamate) Yeast—malt sprout extract	paprika spices turmeric (oleo resin) vanilla, vanillin	annotto extract beta-apo-8' carotenal beta carotene canthaxanthin caramel carrot oil citrus red #2* cochineal extract corn endosperm dehydrated beets dried algae meal FD&C colors* (blue #1, red #3, red #40, yellow #5) grape skin extract iron oxide paprika riboflavin saffron tageles (Aztec Marigold) titanium dioxide toasted, partially defatted, cooked cottonseed flour turmeric (oleo resin) ultramarine blue	corn syrup dextrose fructose glucose invert sugar mannitol saccharin* sorbitol sucrose

turizers, thickeners, leavening agents, dough conditioners, humectants, anti-caking and pH-control agents) are used for food promotion purposes by catering to the consumer's desire for convenience and aesthetic appeal.

- There are questionable risks—minimal at most—associated with the use of certain food additives.
- The choice is yours: It is up to you to evaluate the possible risks and probable benefits associated with the use of food additives.

So, be careful not to over-restrict your intake of either additives or foods! After all, a well-balanced diet which includes a wide variety of nutritious foods should be as enjoyable as it is healthy. Use some common sense and your nutrition know-how in order to make your diet as delicious as it is nutritious.

Aid in Processing or Preparation

Emulsifiers—improve consistency, stability, texture	Stabilizers, Texturizers, Thickeners—give body, improve texture and consistency	Leavening Agents—affect texture and volume	PH-control Agents—change or maintain acidity or alkalinity	Humectants—cause moisture retention
carrageenan diglycerides dioctyl sodium sulfosuccinate lecithin monoglycerides polysorbates sorbitan monostearate	ammonium alginate arabinogalactan calcium alginate carrageenan carob bean gum cellulose gelatin guar gum	calcium phosphate sodium aluminum 　sulfate sodium bicarbonate	acetic acid adipic acid citric acid lactic acid phosphates phosphoric acid propylene glycol sodium acetate	glycerine glycerol monostearate sorbitol
Anti-caking Agents—prevent lumping of crystalline or powdered substances	gum arabic gum ghatti karaya gum	*Maturing and Bleaching Agents, Dough Conditioners*—speed up aging and improve baking qualities	sodium citrate tartaric acid	
calcium silicate iron-ammonium citrate mannitol silicon dioxide yellow prussiate of soda	larch gum locust bean gum mannitol modified food starch pectin potassium alginate propylene glycol sodium alginate sodium calcium alginate	acetone peroxide azodicarbonamide benzoyl peroxide calcium bromate hydrogen peroxide potassium bromate sodium stearyl fumarate		

DAY TWENTY-NINE

DIET AND DRUGS

STEP 1: INTERACTIONS DEFINED

Indicate (✔) which of the following combinations you would avoid:

☐ alcohol and sleeping pills
☐ aspirin on an empty stomach
☐ soybeans and thyroid medication

It has long been an accepted fact that the effects of certain drugs can be altered by other drugs. Consumers need to be aware of the potential health problems associated with undesirable drug interactions. Recently, specific food-drug interactions have also begun to be recognized as a source of certain side effects and adverse reactions. It is now known that various medications can alter nutritional status, and that foods may affect the action of certain drugs. In simple terms, diet-drug interactions can be categorized as:

- drug-influenced nutrient reactions—certain medications affect nutritional status
- food-drug interactions—the presence of food affects the rate and extent of absorption and excretion of certain medications.

With some basic information and a bit of common sense, use of required medications can be effective, safe, and well-coordinated with dietary intake.

STEP 2: RECOGNIZING DRUG-INFLUENCED NUTRIENT REACTIONS

A majority of the important drug-influenced nutrient reactions involve an interference with absorption:

- Laxatives may cause loss of important vitamins, minerals, and fats, and can decrease intestinal absorption of sugars.
- Many drugs which lower cholesterol not only

decrease the absorption of cholesterol, but of sugars, vitamin B_{12} and iron as well.
- Antimicrobials, especially neomycin, may decrease the absorption of fat, folic acid, and vitamin B_{12}.
- Stool softeners and Tween 80 (a supposedly inactive ingredient in many liquid drug formulas) can increase the absorption of cholesterol and vitamin A.
- Drugs that injure the lining of the intestine, such as certain cancer treatment medications, may decrease the absorption of sugars, fat, folic acid, and vitamin B_{12}.
- Anticonvulsants and estrogens decrease the absorption of folic acid.
- Alcohol reduces the absorption of folic acid, vitamin B_{12}, and magnesium.

Drugs can also alter nutritional status by affecting appetite through:

- Altered taste sensation—certain drugs, such as penicillamine, can affect the ability to distinguish between different tastes.
- Unpleasant flavor—several liquid medications, including vitamin B-complex liquids, taste unpleasant and may cause nausea and gastrointestinal upset.
- Nausea—several drugs, including certain intestinal gas and urinary retention preparations, and narcotic pain relievers, often produce nausea.
- Salty, bitter flavor—certain medications which contain potassium or bromide can leave a salty, bitter aftertaste which diminishes appetite.
- Increased appetite—certain tranquilizers, anti-anxiety agents, and antidepressants are believed to stimulate appetite, while oral contraceptives may elicit this reaction in susceptible individuals (see Step 4 for more details).

Obviously, consumers need to be aware of the possible nutritional implications associated with a variety of common medications. It is up to you to be aware of the potential side effects and health consequences of drug therapies.

STEP 3: RECOGNIZING FOOD-DRUG INTERACTIONS

By changing the environment of the digestive tract, the presence of food can alter the rate and extent of absorption and excretion of certain drugs. This can result in:

• An increased rate of drug absorption—certain medications should be taken only on an empty stomach in order to increase drug stability and assure more complete absorption; oral penicillin, for example, is most effective when taken at least one or two hours after mealtime.

• A decreased rate of drug absorption—in creating the needed barrier between irritating drugs and the sensitive digestive tract, food can act to slow down drug absorption; tetracycline, iron salts, potassium supplements, and aspirin, for example, should be taken with or immediately following meals.

• An increased extent of drug absorption—when given with meals high in fat content, griseofulvin, an antibiotic used to treat ringworm and athlete's foot, is more completely absorbed; thiamine appears to be better absorbed when taken with cola beverages.

• A decreased extent of drug absorption—certain drugs bind to food components, creating poor drug absorption; tetracycline, iron, salts, and potassium supplements form such complexes when taken with milk and other dairy products. Also, certain drugs can become partially dissolved if mixed with fruit juices, soft drinks, or ice cream; lesser amounts of penicillin G and erythromycin are made available for absorption with such mixing.

• Altered rate of drug excretion—foods which affect the acidity or alkalinity of the urinary tract can alter the rate of excretion of certain drugs, including amphetamines; protein foods, grains, certain nuts, cranberries, plums, and prunes can cause acidic urine, while milk, vegetables, certain nuts, and most fruits lead to an alkaline urine.

Food intake can also alter drug action through the reactions of specific food substances with certain drug components. Undesirable side effects can be produced, for example:

• Monoamine oxidase inhibitors, used to lower blood pressure and for severe depression, react with foods high in tyramine (eg, aged cheese, bananas, broad beans, chocolate, liver, pickled herring, and wine) and can cause increased blood pressure, headaches, nosebleeds, and stroke.

• Anticoagulants can be less effective with a significant intake of green leafy vegetables.

• Thyroid-like drug action can be interrupted by foods which contain goitrins (eg, broccoli, Brussels sprouts, cabbage, cauliflower, kale, kohlrabi, rutabaga, soybeans, turnip).

These are only a few examples of the known food-drug interactions, and the actual scope of these reactions has yet to be defined. However, with an increased awareness of the possible consequences, you can guard against undesirable interactions between diet and drugs.

STEP 4: "THE PILL"

In the following chart, list all medications, physician-prescribed and over-the-counter, which you take on a regular basis. Include the dosage, frequency of intake, and purpose for usage of each drug. You may then want to use the information given in Steps 2 and 3 to discover if your medication intake has any nutritional implications. Your physician or pharmacist can provide you with any further information you may desire concerning your drug and dietary intakes.

Did you include oral contraceptives in the chart? Are you currently on "The Pill"? Many women tend to forget that these daily tablets are real drugs with real side effects.

Oral contraceptives are composed of the synthetic sex steroid hormones estrogen and progesterone which are taken in a combination form popularly known as "The Pill." "The Pill" is not only prescribed for contraceptive purposes, but may also be used for menstrual irregularities, menopausal problems, acne, and hirsutism (excessive facial hair). "The Pill" has a wide range of side effects, especially important because healthy women may use oral contraceptives for extended periods of time. Some possible side effects associated with use of oral contraceptives include:

• nausea
• digestive disturbances
• headache
• fluid retention
• weight gain
• increased susceptibility to vaginal infections
• mood changes
• gallstones
• high blood pressure
• blood clots

The widespread popularity of "The Pill" has uncovered a number of related nutritional implica-

Drug: Brand/Genetic Name	Dose and Frequency	Reason(s) for Use

tions. Women who take oral contraceptives for extended periods of time should be aware of the possible unfavorable effects on nutritional status.

The absorption and utilization of the following nutrients may be affected by the use of oral contraceptives:

• Carbohydrate—the estrogen component of oral contraceptives may lower the body's ability to tolerate sugars; caution is recommended for women who have or are at high risk of developing diabetes.

• Fat and cholesterol—oral contraceptives increase blood levels of cholesterol; heightened risk for developing atherosclerosis has yet to be established, but increased incidence in women who smoke cigarettes and/or are over age 35 has been noted.

• Vitamin B_6—synthetic estrogen may increase the need for this B-complex vitamin; it is believed that the depression common in many oral contraceptive users may be partially due to an inadequate supply of this vitamin.

• Folic acid—oral contraceptives interfere with the absorption of this B-complex vitamin, and long-term use of "The Pill" can contribute to the development of certain anemias.

• Vitamin B_{12}—low blood levels of this B-complex vitamin have been noted in some oral contraceptive users; normal body stores of vitamin B_{12} can last up to three years, but B_{12} supplementation may be necessary to prevent anemia in women who remain on "The Pill" for longer periods.

• Vitamin C—estrogen causes an increased breakdown rate for this vitamin, resulting in decreased blood levels in some oral contraceptive

users; this disturbance is especially noticeable in cigarette smokers.

• Water and sodium—oral contraceptives may cause fluid retention with bloating and water-weight gain; dietary sodium (salt) intake can contribute to the problem.

Oral contraceptive use may decrease the body's need for certain nutrients, including:

• vitamin A   • iron
• calcium   • copper

Further research on the interactions between "The Pill" and the above nutrients, as well as on other dietary components, is currently underway. Therefore, in order to ensure optimal nutritional health while using oral contraceptives, the following guidelines are recommended:

• Avoid an excessive intake of sugar and foods high in sugar, especially if diabetic or prone to diabetes.
• Avoid an excessive intake of foods high in fat and/or cholesterol, especially if over age 35 or if you smoke cigarettes.
• Include foods high in B-complex vitamins and in vitamin C in the diet each day (see Day Five).
• Avoid excessive salt intake, especially if fluids tend to be retained.

Oral contraceptives are relatively new to the drug market, and possible side effects, both immediate and long-term, are still being researched. A diet which is moderate in sugar, fat, cholesterol, and sodium contents, and which includes foods rich in B-vitamins and vitamin C, may prove to be a necessary nutritional safety precaution. However, if you have been undertaking the daily steps outlined in the Nutri-Plan, use of oral contraceptives should not prove to be a threat to your ever-improving nutritional health.

STEP 5: DAY TWENTY-NINE PLAN

On Day Twenty-Nine, continue to follow your weekly menu planner from Day Twenty-Two and to record all of your physical activities in the chart from Day Twenty-Five. Try to keep emotional stress to a minimum, and make sure that your emotional environment—like your diet—is well-balanced. Also, utilize your nutrition know-how in evaluating the use of health foods in your diet to determine if they are worth the cost. Be careful not to over-restrict your intake of either additives or foods!

For Day Twenty-Nine, use the list of those medications you use on a regular basis (see Step 4) and the information provided in Day Twenty-Nine to note any dietary alterations you may need to make. It is probable that, due to the past 28 days of gradual dietary improvements, few changes will be required.

DAY THIRTY
END OF THE MONTH SUMMARY

STEP 1: IS IT OVER NOW?

During the past month, you have become aware of your own eating habits, learned how to modify your behaviors in order to improve your diet, and made the changes necessary to enhance your nutritional status and overall health. You have gained personal insight and developed nutrition know-how on a variety of diet-related issues, including the following:

- balancing the diet—food and beverage intake record
- protein—sources and needs, alternative choices
- carbohydrate—sources and needs, wise food choices
- fat—amounts and kinds of sources, typical needs
- vitamins—sources and needs, overdose and side effects
- minerals—sources and needs, overdose and side effects
- water—sources and needs, beverages with alcohol, caffeine, and sports or diet purposes
- individual dietary influences—likes and dislikes, styles and beliefs, health factors, and nutrition education
- calories—food sources, determination of individual needs
- dietary goals and guidelines—suggested changes for the American diet
- Fruit and Vegetable Group—wise food choices, fiber in diet and health
- Grain Group—wise food choices, fiber in diet and health
- Milk and Cheese Group—wise food choices, associated health dilemmas
- Meat and Alternates Group—wise food choices, associated health dilemmas
- Others Group—fat, sugar, salt, and alcohol in the diet
- weight loss dieting—fads and facts, Nutri-Plan diet plan

- modifying eating behaviors—dietary influences from the past, the environment, and emotions
- nutrition at home—home planning, home improvements, and tips to try at home
- shopping nutritionally—menu plans, shopping lists, food labels, and supermarket strategy
- dining out—wise food choices for restaurants, parties, on-the-job, and special occasions
- nutritious snacks—wise snack habits and suggested recipes
- nutritious menu planning—weekly menu plans
- nutritious recipes—recommended recipes
- anorexia nervosa—diet overdose and associated health problems
- physical activity—associated health improvements, individualized activity plans
- nutrition and behavior—facts and fads about food and mood
- health foods—claims and scientific facts about the "natural" movement
- additives—"good" and "bad"
- diet and drugs—drug-influenced nutrient reactions, food–drug interactions, "The Pill"

Also during the past month, you have conscientiously maintained an accurate food intake record and had the opportunity to further your nutrition knowledge. It is hoped that you have expanded your self-awareness, and have increased your interest and education in the area of nutrition and health.

So, how do you feel? Has your health improved along with your diet? And have you changed your attitude about the important influence of diet on your health? What exactly have you done?

On Day Thirty, carefully review the past twenty-nine Days, the information and suggestions provided by each Day, and the changes you have made in your own habits and patterns. Then ask yourself the following questions:

Yes No

☐ ☐ Have I learned anything of personal importance?

☐ ☐ Have I employed this knowledge in order to improve my diet and overall health?

☐ ☐ Will I extend this new health-promoting lifestyle beyond Day Thirty?

If you are able to honestly answer Yes to all three of the above questions, Nutri-Plan has successfully assisted you in improving your nutrition education, dietary habits, and overall health. Congratulations! And keep up the good-for-you work! Remember, the choice is yours, the responsibility is yours, and the benefits are yours as well.

FINAL STEP: IS IT REALLY OVER?

You have now spent 30 days learning and practicing new health-related behaviors. You have developed new eating habits and incorporated them into your own lifestyle. You are on your way to optimal health and well-being. So, now what? The Nutri-Plan ends with this chapter; do you end there as well? What is your next step? If the Nutri-Plan has achieved the intended goals of enhanced nutritional awareness and ongoing progress toward improved health, then your next step should be obvious:

Continue to Eat Well to be Fit!

Simply because you have finished with the Nutri-Plan, your new dietary behaviors need not be abandoned. You can continue to incorporate the sound nutritional facts you have learned this past month into your daily lifestyle. Remember, the choice is yours. After all, it is your diet, your health, and your life. And if you so desire, the Nutri-Plan can help to improve your diet, enhance your health, and possibly make your life more enjoyable.

A well-balanced diet which includes a variety of foods in moderate amounts can supply you with the essential nutrients your body needs for optimal health and well-being. The Nutri-Plan has taught you how to balance your diet and optimize your health. It is up to you to do so.

*   *   *

SUMMARY UPDATE

As Nutri-Plan goes to press, there are several new-trition issues which are currently "hot":

• Body Setpoint—Current research is investigating the possibility of a "setpoint" for body fat, or a level of fatness that the body strives to maintain. Possibly controlled by fat storage cells, the theory proposes that chemical signals inform the brain when these cells "need" more fat. This hypothesis may explain both the reason behind stubborn weight plateaus (the setpoint has been reached) and dieting binges (the dieter has gone below his or her individual setpoint which triggers an eating response).

• The Cambridge Diet—A very low-calorie diet formula which is sold door-to-door, potential followers of this weight loss fad were warned of dangerous side effects by the Food and Drug Administration and the American Medical Association. Providing only 330 calories per day in supplement form, this diet is *not* recommended by the nutrition and medical communities.

• Eicosapentaenoic acid (EPA)—These "omega-fatty acids" found in salmon and other fish may help to lower the blood levels of cholesterol and fat in both those with elevated amounts and in normal individuals. EPA may also help to reduce blood clotting, so the dietary role of fish is under research.

• National Academy of Science (NAS) Diet-Cancer Report—The NAS Committee on Diet, Nutrition and Cancer recently issued a 400-page report on the current evidence linking diet and cancer. Although still lacking complete substantiation for their conclusions, the report lent further support to the *Dietary Goals*, and included the following suggestions:

1) Reduce total fat intake for all types of fat.
2) Increase intake of whole grains, fruits, and vegetables, especially those high in vitamins C and A (beta-carotene), and the cruciferae family vegetables (broccoli, cabbage, cauliflower).
3) Minimize intake of salt-pickled, salt-cured, and smoked foods.
4) Moderate alcohol intake, especially with cigarette smoking.

• Sodium Labeling—Government agencies, food industries, and consumer groups are debating the inclusion of sodium information on food labels; such labeling—which would include mg of sodium per serving and/or "low"/"reduced"/"moderately low"/"sodium free"—may become mandatory, or might be a voluntary option for those products that currently provide nutrition labeling.

• Bulimia—An eating disorder whose victims gorge themselves with food and then vomit or purge themselves with laxatives, bulimia has become common among young women who are compulsive dieters and/or prone to anorexia nervosa. Currently estimated to affect 15% to 20% of all college coeds, this dangerous disorder can cause serious medical problems and may require psychological counseling. Information and assistance can be obtained from the National Association of

Anorexia Nervosa and Associated Disorders (ANAD), Box 271-P, Highland Park, IL 60035.

• Caffeine in Exercise—Research is underway to determine whether caffeine may help to decrease muscle fatigue and assist in prolonged endurance during strenuous exercise. Effects are not due to the stimulating effects of caffeine, but through the release of fats into the bloodstream (which are used for energy, sparing the limited glycogen stores). Athletes should keep in mind, however, the diuretic effects and other possible drawbacks of caffeine intake.

• "Light" Foods—A loosely interpreted term used to describe foods and beverages which contain less than the typical amount of a certain ingredient (calories, fat, sugar, sodium, alcohol, etc), this term has yet to be legally defined. Everything from chips and beer to ketchup, cake, wine, and frozen entrees now tout the "lite" claim and the inevitable inflated price tag.

APPENDIX A

Nutri-Plan Diet Diary

Day _____

Time Eating Began to Time Eating Ended	Food and Amount	Hunger Rating*	Comments and Personal Feelings

*Key: PH—Physical hunger; EH—Emotional hunger; OH—Outside/environmental hunger

230

Day _____

Time Eating Began to Time Eating Ended	Food and Amount	Hunger Rating*	Comments and Personal Feelings

*Key: PH—Physical hunger; EH—Emotional hunger; OH—Outside/environmental hunger

APPENDIX B

Recommended Dietary Allowances

FOOD AND NUTRITION BOARD, NATIONAL ACADEMY OF SCIENCES–NATIONAL RESEARCH COUNCIL
RECOMMENDED DAILY DIETARY ALLOWANCES,[a] Revised 1980

Designed for the maintenance of good nutrition of practically all healthy people in the U.S.A.

	Age (years)	Weight (kg)	Weight (lb)	Height (cm)	Height (in)	Protein (g)	Vitamin A (µg RE)[b]	Vitamin D (µg)[c]	Vitamin E (mg α-TE)[d]	Vitamin C (mg)	Thiamin (mg)	Riboflavin (mg)	Niacin (mg NE)[e]	Vitamin B-6 (mg)	Folacin (µg)[f]	Vitamin B-12 (µg)	Calcium (mg)	Phosphorus (mg)	Magnesium (mg)	Iron (mg)	Zinc (mg)	Iodine (µg)
Infants	0.0–0.5	6	13	60	24	kg × 2.2	420	10	3	35	0.3	0.4	6	0.3	30	0.5[g]	360	240	50	10	3	40
	0.5–1.0	9	20	71	28	kg × 2.0	400	10	4	35	0.5	0.6	8	0.6	45	1.5	540	360	70	15	5	50
Children	1–3	13	29	90	35	23	400	10	5	45	0.7	0.8	9	0.9	100	2.0	800	800	150	15	10	70
	4–6	20	44	112	44	30	500	10	6	45	0.9	1.0	11	1.3	200	2.5	800	800	200	10	10	90
	7–10	28	62	132	52	34	700	10	7	45	1.2	1.4	16	1.6	300	3.0	800	800	250	10	10	120
Males	11–14	45	99	157	62	45	1000	10	8	50	1.4	1.6	18	1.8	400	3.0	1200	1200	350	18	15	150
	15–18	66	145	176	69	56	1000	10	10	60	1.4	1.7	18	2.0	400	3.0	1200	1200	400	18	15	150
	19–22	70	154	177	70	56	1000	7.5	10	60	1.5	1.7	19	2.2	400	3.0	800	800	350	10	15	150
	23–50	70	154	178	70	56	1000	5	10	60	1.4	1.6	18	2.2	400	3.0	800	800	350	10	15	150
	51+	70	154	178	70	56	1000	5	10	60	1.2	1.4	16	2.2	400	3.0	800	800	350	10	15	150
Females	11–14	46	101	157	62	46	800	10	8	50	1.1	1.3	15	1.8	400	3.0	1200	1200	300	18	15	150
	15–18	55	120	163	64	46	800	10	8	60	1.1	1.3	14	2.0	400	3.0	1200	1200	300	18	15	150
	19–22	55	120	163	64	44	800	7.5	8	60	1.1	1.3	14	2.0	400	3.0	800	800	300	18	15	150
	23–50	55	120	163	64	44	800	5	8	60	1.0	1.2	13	2.0	400	3.0	800	800	300	18	15	150
	51+	55	120	163	64	44	800	5	8	60	1.0	1.2	13	2.0	400	3.0	800	800	300	10	15	150
Pregnant						+30	+200	+5	+2	+20	+0.4	+0.3	+2	+0.6	+400	+1.0	+400	+400	+150	h	+5	+25
Lactating						+20	+400	+5	+3	+40	+0.5	+0.5	+5	+0.5	+100	+1.0	+400	+400	+150	h	+10	+50

[a] The allowances are intended to provide for individual variations among most normal persons as they live in the United States under usual environmental stresses. Diets should be based on a variety of common foods in order to provide other nutrients for which human requirements have been less well defined. See text for detailed discussion of allowances and of nutrients not tabulated. See Table 1 (p. 20) for weights and heights by individual year of age. See Table 3 (p. 29) for suggested average energy intakes.

[b] Retinol equivalents. 1 retinol equivalent = 1 µg retinol or 6 µg β carotene. See text for calculation of vitamin A activity of diets as retinol equivalents.

[c] As cholecalciferol. 10 µg cholecalciferol = 400 IU of vitamin D.

[d] α-tocopherol equivalents. 1 mg d-α tocopherol = 1 α-TE. See text for variation in allowances and calculation of vitamin E activity of the diet as α-tocopherol equivalents.

[e] 1 NE (niacin equivalent) is equal to 1 mg of niacin or 60 mg of dietary tryptophan.

[f] The folacin allowances refer to dietary sources as determined by *Lactobacillus casei* assay after

treatment with enzymes (conjugases) to make polyglutamyl forms of the vitamin available to the test organism.

[g] The recommended dietary allowance for vitamin B-12 in infants is based on average concentration of the vitamin in human milk. The allowances after weaning are based on energy intake (as recommended by the American Academy of Pediatrics) and consideration of other factors, such as intestinal absorption; see text.

[h] The increased requirement during pregnancy cannot be met by the iron content of habitual American diets nor by the existing iron stores of many women; therefore the use of 30–60 mg of supplemental iron is recommended. Iron needs during lactation are not substantially different from those of nonpregnant women, but continued supplementation of the mother for 2–3 months after parturition is advisable in order to replenish stores depleted by pregnancy.

Taken from: *Recommended Dietary Allowances*, Ninth Revised Edition, 1980. National Academy of Sciences, Washington, DC 20418